Psychoanalysis for Children with ADHD

W0234877

In *Psychoanalysis for Children with ADHD*, a group of eminent analysts highlight the positive impact that psychoanalytic work and the clinical space can have on children with Attention Deficit Hyperactivity Disorder.

Thoroughly researched and informed by decades of work in the field, this volume includes contributions from well-known scientists and analysts such as François Gonon and Patrick Landman. Each contribution addresses sensitive and complex issues, including diagnostic criteria, behavioral problems and patterns, pharmacological intervention, ethical implications and the involvement of parents in treatment. Based on empirical data, the contributors offer a well-balanced critique of standardized approaches to ADHD, and make a case for psychoanalysis as an indispensable tool for both the child with ADHD and their caregivers. Throughout, the book shares the importance of the child having a safe space to explain, in their own words, their mind-body experience.

Written in accessible language, this volume will be of interest to all psychoanalysts and psychotherapists working with children, as well as those offering specialized care in a medical or educational setting.

Sébastien Ponnou is a psychoanalyst and professor in educational sciences at the University of Paris 8, France. His research focuses on psychoanalytic studies, clinical practices, mental health issues, medico-social institutions and the training of social workers.

Psychoanalysis for Children with ADHD

Edited by Sébastien Ponnou

With the contributions of:
David Coto
François Gonon
Pascal-Henri Keller
Patrick Landman
Laurence Morel

Foreword by Valeria Sommer-Dupont

Translated from French by Chad Langford and Judith Van Heerswynghels

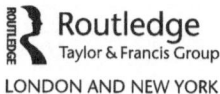

Routledge
Taylor & Francis Group

LONDON AND NEW YORK

Designed cover image: Getty - Anastasiia Sienotova

First published 2025

by Routledge
4 Park Square, Milton Park, Abingdon, Oxon OX14 4RN

and by Routledge
605 Third Avenue, New York, NY 10158

Routledge is an imprint of the Taylor & Francis Group, an informa business

First French edition: 2022 © Champ social;

First English edition published by Routledge 2025

Translated from French by Chad Langford and Judith Van Heerswynghels

ISBN: 978-1-032-95349-6 (hbk)
ISBN: 978-1-032-86314-6 (pbk)
ISBN: 978-1-003-58446-9 (ebk)

DOI: 10.4324/9781003584469

Typeset in Times New Roman
by Deanta Global Publishing Services, Chennai, India

Contents

Index of case studies

Partnership and financial support

The following partners contributed to the funding and publication of this work:

- The University Paris 8 and the Interdisciplinary Research Center on Culture, Education, Training, and Work (CIRCEFT),
- The University of Rouen Normandy and the Interdisciplinary Normand Research Center in Education and Training (CIRNEF),
- The Interdisciplinary Institute for Research in Human and Social Sciences (IRIHS) of Université de Rouen Normandy,
- The Hybrida Social Intervention Scientific Interest Group (GIS Hybrida-IS),
- The Contemporary Institute of Childhood,
- EOVI Mutual Insurance, and the Fondation de l'Avenir for Medical Research.

We sincerely thank them for their contribution to this editorial project.

Contributors

David Coto is a clinical psychologist. He is guided by Freudian psychoanalysis and the teachings of Jacques Lacan and Jacques-Alain Miller. He is particularly interested in the clinic of the child and the adolescent, and in questions related to educational and pedagogical approaches. He works in a medical-educational institution and in a special education and homecare service. He has published several texts in the review *Letterina*: "Ce qui rend nécessaire le symptôme", "Mr. H et le puzzle du monde"; "Clinique d'un trousseau de clefs. The Emerick case"; "Les Choristes ou l'émergence de l'invention et du singulier en institution"; and "Faire écran au regard".

François Gonon is Director of Research Emeritus at the French CNRS (*Centre national de la recherche scientifique*, or National Center for Scientific Research (University of Bordeaux, France)). He worked for 35 years as a neurobiologist and his main work at that time was on neurotransmission involving dopamine. For the last 15 years he has been reorienting his research towards communication sciences. He and his colleagues try to describe the discrepancies between biomedical observations, in particular in psychiatry, and their presentation in the scientific literature and by the media. In this area, he has published a dozen articles in peer-reviewed journals about the media's coverage of ADHD research.

Pascal-Henri Keller is Professor Emeritus at the University of Poitiers, France. He is also a psychoanalyst in Bordeaux and a full member of the Société psychanalytique de Paris. With a dual training as a physiotherapist and psychologist, he has worked in general hospitals and in psychiatric hospitals. His work is partly inspired by this initial professional trajectory. His doctoral thesis in psychology deals with the epistemological foundations of psychosomatics. He has conducted studies on the placebo phenomenon and its uses, as well as on the medicalization of suffering due to depression. For 15 years, he was a member and president of a CPP (Committee for the Protection of Persons) in biomedical research. His publications include Ducousso-Lacaze, A., & Keller, P.-H., 2021, *Ce que les psychanalystes apportent à l'Université*, érès; Keller, P.-H., 2020, *La dépression*, PUF (from the collection *Que sais-je?*) (2nd ed.); Keller, P.-H.,

& Landman, P., 2019, *Ce que les psychanalystes apportent à la société*, érès; Keller, P.-H., & Kreutzer, M., 2018, *Dictionnaire de l'Humain*, ("Instinct"), Presses Universitaires de Nanterre; Keller, P.-H., 2013, *Lettre ouverte au déprimé*, Dunod; Keller, P.-H. (Ed.), 2010, *Le corporel. État des lieux en psychosomatique*, Dunod; Keller, P.-H., 2008, *La question psychosomatique* (from the collection *Topos*), Dunod; and Keller, P.-H., 2006, *Le dialogue du corps et de l'esprit*, Odile Jacob.

Patrick Landman is a psychiatrist, child psychiatrist, psychoanalyst and legal scholar, president of Stop DSM, president of the scientific council of AEVE, former president of Espace Analytique, and author of *Tristesse Business*, published in 2013 by Max Milo, and *Tous hyperactifs*, published in 2016 by Albin Michel.

Laurence Morel is a clinical psychologist, guided by Lacanian psychoanalysis, and a member of the Association de la Cause Freudienne (ACF) in Normandy. She works in the child psychiatry sector in a French CPP (*centre médico-psychologique*, or medical-psychological center). She is in charge of an association which manages the LAEP (or child–parent reception center) in Verneuil d'Avre et d'Iton (the association *Chemins d'enfance*, "Les Petits Pas"). She also works there to help the children and parents who come for support.

Sébastien Ponnou is a psychoanalyst and a member of the École de la Cause Freudienne (ECF) and the World Association of Psychoanalysis (WAP). He is also a professor of educational sciences at Paris 8 University (CIRCEFT EPsyFor – Education, Psychoanalysis, Training – EA 4384). His work focuses on psychoanalytic studies, clinical practices and mental health issues, medico-social institutions and the training of social workers. Sébastien Ponnou leads several research projects on diagnostic and therapeutic challenges in child and adolescent psychiatry, through the analysis of health databases. He is an expert member of the Council for Childhood and Adolescence of the French High Council for Family, Childhood, and Aging (HCFEA). He is also a member of the Association de la Cause Freudienne (ACF) in Normandy. Recent publications (French editions): Ponnou, S. (Ed.). (2025). *Psychoanalysis for Children with Autism*. Nîmes: Champ Social Éditions. Ponnou, S., Briffault, X., & Chave, F. (Eds.). (2023). *The Silence of Symptoms: A Study on Mental Health and Child Care*. Nîmes: Champ Social Éditions. Ponnou, S. (Ed.). (2022). *Psychoanalysis for ADHD Children*. Nîmes: Champ Social Éditions.

Valeria Sommer-Dupont is a psychologist, a psychoanalyst and a member of the École de la Cause Freudienne (ECF) and of the World Association of Psychoanalysis (WAP). She coordinates the Centre d'Étude et de Recherche sur l'Enfant dans le Discours Analytique (or Center for Study and Research on the Child in Analytical Discourse (New Network CEREDA)).

Translators

Chad Langford is an independent translator based in the north of France. He is head of Foreign Language Teaching for Continuing Studies at the Center for Languages (CLIL DELANG) at the University of Lille. He is the co-author of *Advanced English Grammar: A Linguistic Approach* published by Bloomsbury, soon in its third edition.

Judith Van Heerswynghels taught translation at the University of Lille, where she was in charge of the Masters in subtitling. Her translation of a collection of short stories and poetry by Rudyard Kipling appears in Gallimard's La Pléiade collection.

Langford and Van Heerswynghels are frequent collaborators.

Foreword

Valeria Sommer-Dupont

The function of psychoanalysts is not self-evident, nor is their place in the world. This place is acquired, says Lacan, by pushing and shoving your way into it.

We do not choose our jobs randomly, but there is indeed something random about the choices we make. The aim of an analysis is for us to know something about why we do one job rather than another, why we have become part of a certain professional lineage, and also why – and how – we choose to use a given discourse to explain and perform our work.

Knowing something of the discourse that sustains us and that we then maintain, of the way in which we embody it and allow it to exist, is a necessary condition for becoming an analyst. The Lacanian lexicon has a concept for this, *the desire of the psychoanalyst*: "[the] desire of the psychoanalyst[s] [...] neither obeys rules nor follows a technique, but presupposes that the analysts have done work on themselves that enables them to grasp the way in which their desire is absorbed in psychoanalysis" (Lacan, 1970, p. 19). Being clear about one's own discourse and the way in which it is given substance is central to psychoanalytic practice. Within the framework of this discourse, analysts do not allow themselves to do this job without endeavoring to *decenter*, a process which consists in analyzing how psychoanalysts become part of the whole picture.

During a conference in Bordeaux in 1968, Lacan pointed out the *contemporaneity* between two discursive facts, that of psychoanalysis and the fact that science alone has something to tell us (Lacan, 2005, p. 97). Since this relation of contemporaneity was put forward by Lacan, it follows that there is an urgent need to establish the criteria for delineating a logical and ethical *non-relation of structure*. The articles in this volume, edited by Sébastien Ponnou, show that, almost 60 years later, it is still necessary to insist upon this difference. Psychoanalysis does not deny the existence of the brain, neurons or genes. Indeed, it developed at the same time as the scientific "advances" related to them. What psychoanalysis *does* want to make clear is that these things have nothing to do with the unconscious and that the notion of "progress", an article of faith which scientism blindly espouses, must be used with caution.

That a discourse uses signifiers to name what it claims to treat does not surprise us: "ADHD", "intellectual giftedness", "precocious child", and all the terms that begin with the prefix "dys-" (such as dysgraphia, dysorthography or dyspraxia) are signifiers in the same way as the terms "neurosis", "psychosis" and "perversion". The difference lies elsewhere.

On the one hand, those who use psychoanalytic discourse posit the unconscious as a hypothesis and assume that words are signifiers. At the same time, they maintain that a signifier is fundamentally insignificant and that, as analysts, they are "in the know". On the other hand, science advocates hypostasizing the diagnosis and the diagnosed reality, stripping all signifying value from the words they use to refer to this reality that they claim to examine from afar.

As the offspring of two discourses, that of a certain science and that of capitalism, the science advocate rejects both *hystory*[1] and the origin of the diagnosis. For him, the diagnosis is a thing *in and of itself*, independent and autonomous, a pure and simple objective fact wandering in what he calls a *natural nature*, separate from the subjective world, which is considered vague and related to humans. Science advocates conceive, while conveniently "forgetting" that it is only a "conception". They see the diagnosis as having objectifiable, measurable, locatable, visible and tangible causes. They conceive it, while "forgetting" that they are the ones who conceive it. Science advocates construct the instruments that will allow them to objectify, measure, locate, see and touch, "forgetting" that "if one questions a child from the logical apparatus of the interrogator [...] one should not be surprised to find it in the person being questioned" (Lacan, 2005, p. 47). They construct the experiment, while "forgetting" that they too are part of the picture. Their aim is to reign as the possessors of knowledge about the real. The truth thus obtained is nothing more than a question-begging inference.

The contributions in this volume allow us to grasp the significance of what Lacan says in his seminar on *Les Quatre Concepts fondamentaux de la psychanalyse*: "The status of the unconscious, which I indicate to you as being so fragile on the ontic level, is ethical" (Lacan, 1973, p. 34). Those who use psychoanalytic discourse cannot ignore the *fragility of the unconscious on the ontic level*. As for origin, place and end, Lacan never ceases to remind us that "[e]xperience is only constituted as such if it starts from a correct question. We call this a hypothesis. [...] Something has begun to take the form of a fact, and a fact is always made up of discourse" (Lacan, 2005, p. 92). The unconscious is only a hypothesis, meaning that its contingent existence depends on a simple desiring being: there must be at least one, one *parlêtre*, who posits the unconscious as existence, and he or she must believe in it.

One might think that considering the unconscious to be a hypothesis and psychoanalysis to be a discourse among others would make this practice less "true" or less "real". Quite the opposite is true. Asserting that psychoanalysis is only one discourse among others brings us back to the question of choice, and therefore to the ethical question: why the unconscious? Why choose psychoanalysis to listen to so-called hyperactive children? In this volume, Sébastien Ponnou shares his committed answer with us and invites each contributing author to do the same. This is not an ontological question, but a true ethical one.

Note

1 In the Preface to the English edition of *Séminaire XI*, Lacan creates the neologism *hystory* as a combination of the words "history" and "hysteria", thus asserting a link between saying and truth. In the 14 December 1976 lesson from his seminar *L'insu que sait de l'une bévue s'aile à mourre*, Lacan speaks of *hystoric*, including in this neologism a third term, the "torus": a topological figure with which Lacan approaches the *living body* (Lacan, 1976–1977).

References

Lacan, J. (1970). Discours à l'E.F.P., 6 décembre 1967. *Scilicet*, (2–3), 9–29.

Lacan, J. (1973). *Le Séminaire*, vol. XI: *Les Quatre Concepts fondamentaux de la psychanalyse*. Text established by J.-A. Miller. Paris: Seuil.

Lacan J. (1976–1977). Le Séminaire, livre XXIV, L'insu que sait de l'une-bévue s'aile à mourre. Unpublished.

Lacan, J. (2005). *Mon Enseignement*. Paris: Seuil.

Introduction

Sébastien Ponnou

Attention Deficit Disorder with or without Hyperactivity (ADHD) is considered the most common mental disorder in school-age children. ADHD children are restless, anxious, troubled, turbulent, inattentive and hyperactive. ADHD has become a part of our contemporary real. It is a major public health issue as well as a genuine social phenomenon.

For all that, ADHD is not a psychoanalytical category. This does not stem from ignorance or neglect. Rather, it is because psychoanalysis is an uncategorized practice, a practice of the infinitely specific wherein there exists no common yardstick to evaluate human beings. An analyst takes in the child's suffering, symptoms and words. This is not to say that they disregard or underestimate nosographic aspects, but that they rely first and foremost on the immeasurable value of the child's words and those of his or her parents, beyond any diagnostic or classificatory goal. This is a general fact: the analyst is interested in the child before and beyond his or her disorder, before and beyond any pathology or disability. Analysts aim to reveal the absolute difference of each individual. They support the novelty of a subjective stance and the inventiveness of what emerges from the encounter. The fact that hyperactivity, inattention or ADHD are terms on which specialists rely to treat these children is in no way contradictory to the practice or ethics of psychoanalysis, hence the interest and benefit of the analytical clinic in complex psychological, social and family situations.

It follows that the words of children and of their parents are infinitely more valuable to the analyst than any measurement scale or diagnostic manual, all the more so as international scientific research does not favor biomedical and standardized approaches to hyperactivity.

The limits of biomedical approaches to ADHD

ADHD has been the subject of thousands of studies internationally, the result being that our scientific knowledge of it has increased considerably over the past several decades. Initial studies in the 1980s and 1990s aimed to identify neurological and genetic factors for ADHD with an eye to developing a reliable biological test for the

DOI: 10.4324/9781003584469-1

disorder. At the same time, these same studies aimed to demonstrate that psycho-stimulant drug treatments were effective for ADHD. However, more than 30 years later, no biological factor has been identified for ADHD, and the biological hypotheses initially put forward in the literature have all been refuted. Moreover, as brain imaging and genetic sequencing techniques advance, the likelihood of identifying biological factors for ADHD is decreasing (Gaugler et al., 2014; Gizer, Ficks, & Waldman, 2009; Gonon, 2009; Shaw et al., 2007; Li et al., 2014; Ponnou & Gonon, 2017; Gonon, Dumas-Mallet, & Ponnou, 2019; Ponnou, Haliday, & Gonon, 2020). There are also other aspects to consider. Drug prescription can be useful to support the child's work with words (within the framework of Lacanian psychoanalysis; see Golse & Zigante, 2002) as well as therapeutic, educational and social measures that can underpin care pathways. However, studies carried out over many years show that psychostimulant treatments do not improve the academic performance of children diagnosed with ADHD. Furthermore, these treatments do not reduce the risks of delinquency or addiction associated with hyperactivity (Currie, Stabile, & Jones, 2014; Gonon, Guilé, & Cohen, 2010; Humphreys, Eng, & Lee, 2013; Loe & Feldman, 2007; Sharpe, 2014; The MTA Cooperative Group, 1999).

The contributions presented in this volume provide an enlightened and well-argued critical take on biomedical approaches to hyperactivity/ADHD. In each case, these clinical studies advocate psychoanalytical practices for children or adolescents diagnosed with hyperactivity and their families.

The benefits of psychoanalysis

The aim of this volume is to highlight how psychoanalysts focus on the words of each individual child and those of his or her parents, irrespective of any categorial, deterministic or normative aspect.

Given this, psychoanalysis is understood as what operates in the epiphany of the encounter between the child and the analyst. Moreover, the concepts and the analytical posture have long since gone beyond the sole framework of the cure to support the work carried out in schools and in medico-social institutions. In this sense, psychoanalysis occupies an important place in care and education practices insofar as it is the only approach to be based exclusively on the dimension of transference and to build on the symptoms, resistances and stumbling blocks that signal the existence of the unconscious and of *jouissance*.

Guided by Freud's discovery and innovation and by the teachings of Jacques Lacan and Jacques-Alain Miller, this volume aims to show the effects of psychoanalysis in the care of children and adolescents diagnosed as hyperactive. The emphasis is on individual cases, the inventions and words of the subject and meaning or non-meaning that emerge during sessions with psychoanalysts and within various institutional entities. These are the clinical issues at the heart of practices making use of transference.

This volume brings together contributions from psychoanalysts or practitioners influenced by psychoanalysis. These contributions can account for the phenomenon of displacement and opening at work in sessions with ADHD children. The clinical cases presented here deal with the care of children in a private practice or in an institution and – via the question of hyperactivity – favor the emergence or the development of questions specific to psychoanalysis, including speech and the body, the use of categories and diagnostic references in psychoanalysis, the place of medicinal treatment, working with parents and the ethics of psychoanalysis.

But let us not be mistaken: this volume is not only about psychoanalysis or psychoanalysts; it is above all for parents and for all those involved in care, education and social intervention who are influenced by the practice of listening and speaking, the transmission of knowledge and the helping of others. It is for those who give priority to the voice of the child and his or her parents rather than to diagnostic evaluation grids and who prefer the therapeutic or educational relationship to standardized protocols and practices. This collection is also for those who are not satisfied with deterministic judgements and ready-made solutions, and who every day support, in their practice, in their commitment and in their physical presence, the case-by-case work and the unexpected and unprecedented events which define the depth of clinical practices (Ponnou & Niewiadomski, 2022). Finally, this collection is for politicians and public authorities, in order to alert them to the distortions and conflicts of interest that plague contemporary scientific discourse on the issue of hyperactivity/ADHD. These biases and networks of influence are widely revealed and proven throughout this volume, insofar as they contribute to masking the diversity and specificity of a culturally ingrained form of speech-based psychological care, both of which are well established in the clinic and are the mark of French psychiatry and psychopathology.

Organization of the volume

The collection opens with a text by **François Gonon**, neurobiologist and Director of Research Emeritus at the CNRS, who specializes in dopamine neurotransmitters, ADHD and the discourse of neuroscience. In a chapter entitled "**The scientific discourse on ADHD: evolution, critical analysis and questions**", the author offers an informed critique of the scientific debates on hyperactivity. Starting with a historical approach to the names given to ADHD, he presents the biases inherent in the representations of this pathology in biomedical research and in the media. It then discusses the effects of these distortions for the clinician, in terms of both diagnosis and therapy. The chapter concludes with a critique of the concept of neurodevelopmental disorder and an argument for taking social and environmental factors into account in supporting children diagnosed with ADHD and their families.

The second chapter of the book, entitled "**Listening to children rather than to the sirens of scientism**", is written by **Patrick Landman**, psychiatrist, child psychiatrist and psychoanalyst. Starting from a discussion bringing together psychiatry, science and scientism, the author levels a meticulous critique of the different biomedical hypotheses concerning hyperactivity/ADHD in the scientific literature. Faced with the temptation of scientism and the risk of denying the psychological suffering that can result from it, Patrick Landman advocates a sensitive clinic, marked by nuance and delicacy. The author shows the radical change that took place when André, who had been tested, diagnosed and medicated many times, started seeing him in the context of an analysis. The practices of listening and speaking became the logical and clinical operators contributing to the care of the child and the support of his parents. The presentation also shows the particular use that can be made of medicinal treatment together with listening to the child's words.

In "**The problem with biomedical approaches and the necessity for psychoanalysis as exemplified by hyperactivity/ADHD**", Sébastien Ponnou – psychoanalyst and senior lecturer at the University of Paris 8 – addresses the results of a series of studies dedicated to the prevalence, medication and representations of ADHD in France over the last ten years. He discusses the inexorable increase in the prescription of psychostimulants in children and adolescents, the systematic undermining of prescription regulations, the academic and social factors of diagnosis and medication, and the risk of substituting psychotherapeutic and socio-educational practices with medicinal practices. Faced with these observations, the author denounces the scientific bias, media bias and conflicts of interest that influence the demands, practices and policies of care for children and their families. These reflections highlight the importance of educational, preventive and social support practices, but above all the necessity of psychoanalysis and its clinic in helping the suffering child and his or her parents.

The following chapter is by **Pascal-Henri Keller**, psychoanalyst and Professor Emeritus of Psychology at the University of Poitiers. In his text "**The hyperactive child, an unusual collective myth**", Pascal-Henri Keller discusses Bradley and Wallon's work on the theme of the turbulent child. Denouncing the representations of the "behavioral child" and the medicalization of human behavior, the author proposes a clinical presentation in a private practice – the case of Jordy – in order to bring clarity to the debate, adopting a clinical and theoretical point of view. It shows the analyst's attention to the family history and to the child's words, and his interest in the unexpected elements that emerge through the nightmares that Jordy evokes during the sessions and that will form the framework of his treatment.

In a chapter entitled "**ADHD: from disorder to individual invention**", clinical psychologist **David Coto** testifies to the rich contribution of clinical practices influenced by psychoanalysis in institutions. Starting from an interpretation of *zapping* as a contemporary modality of pleasure and social bonding, the author supports a practice without standards, but not without principles, where invention is the norm. There are four clinical presentations in this invaluable text: it accurately reflects how demanding this work can be in the context of an institution, a kind of work in which words and the body are interwoven. Coto focuses on the details and on the infinite individualities that emerge in psychoanalytic encounters. He invents the devices and working methods that are closest to the subject's words.

In "**Anastasia: a new choreography**", clinical psychologist **Laurence Morel** relates the long-term care and follow-up of Anastasia and her parents. In this clinical account of rare density, Laurence Morel shows to what extent the child's agitation is part of her history and psychological life. It is a symptom of a traumatic reality that is revealed in the work with words and in nightmares. The child ultimately finds peace within the space of the analytical encounter. Beyond the instances of *bon-heurt* (or blessings in disguise) and the discoveries that mark out the child's journey, this text allows us to grasp the importance of the analyst's presence and desire, and of her particular interest in the child. The reader will also appreciate the constancy and delicacy of Morel's interventions, whose pause points, nuances and deviations allow Anastasia to seize her creative opportunity in her relationship with others, with knowledge and with social relationships.

Finally, in a last chapter entitled **"Franck: a case of ADHD"**, **Sébastien Ponnou** presents a clinical case in an institutional context. This contribution sheds new light on the underlying theory specific to the Lacanian approach to hyperactivity.

References

Currie, J., Stabile, M., & Jones, L. (2014). Do stimulant medications improve educational and behavioral outcomes for children with ADHD? *Journal of Health Economics, 37,* 58–69.

Gaugler, T., Klei, L., Sanders, S. J., Bodea, C. A., Goldberg, A. P., Lee, A. B., ... Buxbaum, J. D. (2014). Most genetic risk for autism resides with common variation. *Nature Genetics, 46*(8), 881–885.

Gizer, I. R., Ficks, C., & Waldman, I. D. (2009). Candidate gene studies of ADHD: A meta-analytic review. *Human Genetics, 126*(1), 51–90.

Golse, B., & Zigante, F. (2002). L'enfant, les psychotropes et la psychanalyse. *Revue française de psychanalyse, 66*(2), 433–446.

Gonon, F. (2009). The dopaminergic hypothesis of attention-deficit/hyperactivity disorder needs re-examining. *Trends in Neurosciences, 32*(1), 2–8.

Gonon, F., Dumas-Mallet, E., & Ponnou, S. (2019). La couverture médiatique des observations scientifiques concernant les troubles mentaux. *Les Cahiers du journalisme, 2*(3), R45–R63.

Gonon, F., Guilé, J. M., & Cohen, D. (2010). Le trouble déficitaire de l'attention avec hyperactivité: données récentes des neurosciences et de l'expérience nord-américaine. *Neuropsychiatrie de l'enfance et de l'adolescence, 58*(5), 273–281.

Humphreys, K. L., Eng, T., & Lee, S. S. (2013). Stimulant medication and substance use outcomes: A meta-analysis. *JAMA Psychiatry, 70*(7), 740–749.

Li, Z., Chang, S. H., Zhang, L. Y., Gao, L., & Wang, J. (2014). Molecular genetic studies of ADHD and its candidate genes: A review. *Psychiatry Research, 219*(1), 10–24.

Loe, I., & Feldman, H. (2007). Academic and educational outcomes of children with ADHD. *Journal of Pediatric Psychology, 32*(6), 643–654.

The MTA Cooperative Group. (1999). Moderators and mediators of treatment response for children with attention-deficit/hyperactivity disorder. *Archives of General Psychiatry, 56*(12), 1088–1096.

Ponnou, S., & Gonon, F. (2017). How French media have portrayed ADHD to the lay public and to social workers. *International Journal of Qualitative Studies on Health and Well-Being, 12*(sup1), 1298244.

Ponnou, S., Haliday, H., & Gonon, F. (2020). Where to find accurate information on attention-deficit hyperactivity disorder? A study of scientific distortions among French websites, newspapers, and television programs. *Health (London)*, *24*(6), 684–700.

Ponnou, S., & Niewiadomski, C. (Eds.). (2022). *Critical Psychoanalytic Social Work: Research and Case Studies for Clinical Practice*. New York: Taylor & Francis.

Sharpe, K. (2014). Medication: The smart-pill oversell. *Nature*, *506*(7487), 146–148. https://www.nature.com/news/medication-the-smart-pill-oversell-1.14701

Shaw, P., Gornick, M., Lerch, J., Addington, A., Seal, J., Greenstein, D., … & Rapoport, J. L. (2007). Polymorphisms of the dopamine D4 receptor, clinical outcome, and cortical structure in attention-deficit/hyperactivity disorder. *Archives of General Psychiatry*, *64*(8), 921–931.

Chapter 1

The scientific discourse on ADHD: evolution, critical analysis and questions

François Gonon

***

1. Introduction

To point out that science is not an opinion, but rather a form of discourse, is to bestow on it a great honor. Scientific discourse has its unspoken rules, such as clearly separating the description of observations from subsequent interpretation. It is guided by an ethic: to describe things and living beings as closely as possible to what one believes to be accurate. Above all, it has a goal: to make contradictory debate among researchers possible. Any scientific article is an element of this discourse and immediately becomes part of this debate since it recalls the state of knowledge already published on the subject before proposing an interpretation of new observations in light of previous publications. Scientific knowledge is therefore a cumulative process made possible by the open exchange of rational arguments.

Scientific discourse has a history. It is influenced by conflicts of interest and passing fads as well as by the personal opinions of researchers and their failures. The reflections put forth in this contribution are based on my 15 years of experience as an academic researcher in the analysis of scientific discourse regarding psychiatry and ADHD in particular. I invite the reader to bear in mind that I have no clinical experience with mental disorders and that this necessarily limits the scope of my reflections.

2. Some historical milestones

2.1. The evolution of terminology

Symptoms of ADHD in children were identified as early as the 19th century, particularly excessive inattention and agitation (Mahone & Denckla, 2017; Martinez-Badía & Martinez-Raga, 2015; Smith, 2017; Wolraich et al., 2019). Consistent with the psychiatry of the time, these symptoms were attributed to a

DOI: 10.4324/9781003584469-2

weakness of character that could be due to either a brain injury or a combination of hereditary and environmental factors (Wolraich et al., 2019). Throughout the 20th century, and until the publication of DSM-III in 1980, childhood hyperactivity syndrome was often included in the category of disorders due to minimal brain damage or minimal brain dysfunction, depending on the authors (Mahone & Denckla, 2017; Wolraich et al., 2019). The link between ADHD symptoms and minor brain damage had been suggested by analogy with similar behaviors observed in some children with encephalitis (Wolraich et al., 2019). However, by the late 1970s, the lack of evidence of brain damage had led to the abandonment of this term, suggesting a neurological etiology for more neutral terms (e.g. *hyperkinetic syndrome*). At the same time, Canadian psychologists showed that attention deficit was most often observed in hyperactive children with a normal intelligence quotient (Campbell et al., 1971).

With the introduction of DSM-III in 1980, which was meant to be atheoretical, these same psychologists gained influence, resulting in the definition of Attention Deficit Disorder (Lange et al., 2010; Wolraich et al., 2019). The 1987 revision of DSM-III specified that attention deficit may or may not be associated with hyperactivity, resulting in the current terminology: Attention-Deficit/Hyperactivity Disorder (ADHD) (Wolraich et al., 2019).

Finally, DSM-V, published in 2013, created the group of neurodevelopmental disorders which include ADHD, autism spectrum disorders and learning disabilities. The term "neurodevelopmental disorder" means that these disorders occur in childhood and that the diagnostic boundaries between them are not clear, since comorbidities are common (Thapar et al., 2017). According to its advocates, this term also implies that neurodevelopmental disorders are lifelong conditions and not episodic disorders (Thapar et al., 2017). Thus, adult ADHD would simply be a continuation of childhood ADHD. However, experts acknowledge that "different neurodevelopmental disorders are highly heterogeneous in terms of clinical features, etiology and treatment" (Thapar et al., 2017). In other words, there are no common biological features to support the creation of a category that, furthermore, does little to help the clinician to choose an appropriate treatment (Thapar et al., 2017).

2.2. The treatment of ADHD with psychostimulants

The beneficial effect of amphetamine derivatives on the behavior of agitated children was discovered in 1937. Methylphenidate was first marketed in 1954 as an antidepressant under the name *Ritalin*®. During the 1960s it became apparent that methylphenidate was as effective as amphetamine in improving the symptoms in hyperactive children, particularly their behavior in school, but that it had fewer adverse side effects (Campbell et al., 1971). However, until the mid-1980s the prescription of methylphenidate in children remained marginal, even in the USA. The pharmaceutical industry showed little interest in it since Ritalin was no longer under patent.

In 1980, the pharmaceutical company Ciba-Geigy patented a delayed-release form of methylphenidate (Ritalin-SR) which was authorized for prescription to ADHD children in the USA in 1982. From 1987 onwards, the American association CHADD (*Children and Adults with ADD*), supported by Ciba-Geigy, campaigned for the recognition of ADHD as a disability, which would entitle concerned parties to financial compensation. In 1990, the Supreme Court imposed less restrictive standards for mental disability on the US federal government. As a result of this regulatory change, the number of American children diagnosed with ADHD and treated with a psychostimulant increased fivefold in the space of ten years (Mayes et al., 2008). During the last two decades, this increase has continued, albeit at a slower rate, in the USA, but also in all developed countries (Raman et al., 2018). However, there are significant differences in prescription rates between countries (Raman et al., 2018) and, within countries, between regions (Smith, 2017). For example, in the USA the rate of prescribing a medication for ADHD to children aged 4–17 years varied between 2% in Nevada and 10.4% in Louisiana in 2011 (Visser et al., 2014).

In the short and medium term (14 months), medication reduces ADHD symptoms in 75% of children diagnosed with ADHD (The MTA Cooperative Group, 1999). However, academic difficulties, which appear starting in primary school, are the main reason behind the diagnosis of ADHD. Diagnosed children very clearly perform less well in school than their peers (Baweja et al., 2015). Treatment with psychostimulants improves the academic productivity of ADHD children in the short term, but not the quality of their work (Baweja et al., 2015; Prasad et al., 2013). In terms of population, moreover, the effect on school performance appears to be non-existent or at best insignificant and comes nowhere close to bridging the achievement gap between diagnosed and undiagnosed children (Baweja et al., 2015; Jangmo et al., 2019; Sharpe, 2014).

2.3. The recent evolution of neurobiology

The dramatic increase in the number of children diagnosed with ADHD in the USA has been followed, with a delay of about five years, by an increase in the number of scientific articles about ADHD. Indeed, from 1985 to 1995 this number increased from 195 to 280 while it reached 2,179 in 2015 (according to PubMed). Our purpose here is not to report on these studies in detail, but rather to summarize some of their conclusions. First, it should be noted that none of these studies have proved the existence of a biological marker for ADHD or led to the discovery of a new drug. Studies in genetics targeting dopaminergic neurotransmission looked very promising in the 1990s but have since been invalidated by subsequent studies. Whole-genome studies have shown that ADHD, like other psychiatric disorders, is associated with many frequent polymorphisms, each of which contributes only marginally to the disorder. Moreover, these polymorphisms are rarely specific and are also found in other mental disorders. According to some researchers, the measurement of a polymorphism score associated with ADHD could one day reach a predictive value, but this is not yet the case (Thapar, 2018).

Similarly, the increase in brain imaging studies has not made it possible to reliably identify structural or functional abnormalities in patients. Two very large reviews, one of them written by one of the pioneers of ADHD brain imaging, Xavier Castellanos, have indeed pointed out that findings from different studies diverge (Cortese et al., 2021; Samea et al., 2019).

2.4.   Environmental risks

The large number of studies on genetic abnormalities associated with ADHD can be accounted for by the fact that ADHD is clearly more common in certain families. Family studies, or studies comparing identical and fraternal twins, have found a heritability rate of ADHD of 75% (Hinshaw, 2018). This high rate is often misinterpreted as evidence that ADHD is a genetic disease. However, experts are prompt to point out that high heritability rates in no way exclude the importance of environmental risks: the measure of heritability takes into account the correlations between genes, the environment and their interactions (Hinshaw, 2018; Thapar & Cooper, 2016).

Preterm birth and low birth weight are two risk factors for the subsequent development of ADHD (Galera et al., 2011; Hinshaw, 2018). These risks, often linked, are in part socially determined, as the preterm birth rate is 6% in France and 13% in the USA (Goldenberg et al., 2008). Exposure in utero and during childhood to various toxicants such as lead is also a risk factor (Hinshaw, 2018; Thapar & Cooper, 2016). Other factors have been clearly associated with ADHD, including abuse in early childhood, having a teenage or depressed mother, and poverty (Galera et al., 2011; Hinshaw, 2018).

Other social and institutional factors are rarely taken into account. For example, excessive exposure to screens is a risk factor that is all the more worrying given its rapid increase (Tamana et al., 2019; Weiss et al., 2011). The diagnosis of ADHD is also strongly linked to the year a child enters primary school. In countries where children enter primary school according to their year of birth, the youngest children (i.e. in France, those born in December) are twice as often diagnosed with ADHD as the oldest (i.e. in France, those born in January of the same year) (Whitely et al., 2019). On the contrary, this phenomenon is not observed in Denmark, where initial admission to primary school takes into account the child's maturity (Whitely et al., 2019). Finally, in the USA, there are significant differences in the prescribing of psychostimulants to children. These are largely explained by disparities in public school funding (Fulton et al., 2015): the states with the highest prevalence are those that condition this funding on student achievement and allow teachers to recommend ADHD diagnosis to parents (Fulton et al., 2015).

3. Critical analysis of the scientific discourse on ADHD

3.1. An example: the volume of subcortical structures in ADHD patients

In 2017, Hoogman et al. published a study in *Lancet Psychiatry* that they presented as the largest study to date on the volume of subcortical structures in patients diagnosed with ADHD. According to the authors, their results "confirm that the brains of ADHD patients are altered, providing evidence that ADHD is indeed a brain disease" (Hoogman, Bralten et al., 2017). Of all the cortical structures measured in this study, the one that showed the greatest difference in volume between ADHD patients and controls was the amygdala. On average, the volume of the amygdala in patients is 1.5% smaller than in controls while the standard deviation among controls and patients is 9.5% (Hoogman, Bralten et al., 2017). In other words, approximately 40% of ADHD patients have a greater amygdala volume than the average control, and 40% of controls have a smaller volume than the average patient. Since the amygdala plays a major role in emotion management, the authors conclude that emotion regulation is defective in patients diagnosed with ADHD. This regulation deficit is not included in the DSM-V list of ADHD symptoms, although it is frequently observed (Hinshaw, 2018). Finally, note that the structural differences reported by Hoogman et al. were not confirmed by a more recent meta-analysis (Samea et al., 2019).

In concluding that ADHD is a brain disease, Hoogman et al. added that ADHD is therefore not due to poor parenting. This statement is in contradiction with epidemiological studies showing that maltreatment and excessive exposure to screens are risk factors for ADHD. When the press reported on this study, the causal relationship between these volume differences and ADHD was made even more explicit. Thus, the *Daily Telegraph* of 16 February 2017 headlined: "ADHD is a brain disorder, not a label for poor parenting" (Bodkin, 2017). In the same article it was also stated that "the researchers who carried out the study say their findings prove for the first time that the condition does have a physical cause".

Commenting on the study by Hoogman et al., researchers pointed out that such minor volume differences could as easily be the consequence of ADHD as the cause: correlation is not causality. They regretted that the media asserted the existence of this causal link, thus spreading "a misleading message" (Batstra et al., 2017). To this critical comment, Hoogman et al. replied that they had never established a causal link and that they were in no way responsible for the media's misrepresentations (Hoogman, Buitelaar et al., 2017).

3.2. Distortions of the discourse present in the scientific literature

Numerous academic studies have described and quantified the different forms of discourse distortion in scientific literature. Two recent reviews have synthesized these studies on biomedical research in general (Boutron & Ravaud, 2018; West

& Bergstrom, 2021), and two others have focused on psychiatry (Dumas-Mallet & Gonon, 2020; Gonon et al., 2019). I will briefly describe the different forms of distortion below.

- *Publication bias*: Researchers prefer to publish positive results to the detriment of observations showing no difference between patients and control groups or showing no effect of a treatment, for example. A consequence of this bias is that the first publication on a new question more often reports a positive effect than subsequent studies on the same question. This phenomenon has been observed in the case of ADHD studies (Dumas-Mallet et al., 2016; Gonon et al., 2012).
- *Embellished results*: Results are often presented in such a way as to appear more positive than they really are. Several embellishment procedures can be described: the arbitrary elimination of negative observations; the deliberate choice of a statistical test that confirms the researchers' hypotheses; the omission of methodological information questioning the relevance of the observations; and an abstract presenting observations that are biased or even in conflict with those reported in the article. In particular, cases of embellishment have been reported in the scientific literature concerning ADHD (Gonon et al., 2011b, 2019).
- *Biased interpretation*: The most misleading way to present data is to suggest a causal link on the basis of observations that show only a correlation. For ADHD, the example given above illustrates this interpretation bias (see also Gonon & Cohen, 2011 for another example). The promise of a new treatment for humans based solely on observations in laboratory rats is another form of biased interpretation that has been described for ADHD (Gonon et al., 2011a).
- *Citation bias*: Researchers prefer to cite positive results and those in agreement with their hypotheses and to ignore those that contradict them (Dumas-Mallet et al., 2021). For example, the French National Authority for Health (*Haute Autorité de Santé*) published a recommendation in December 2014 concerning ADHD. The scientific rationale of this recommendation asserts that prescribing psychostimulants to ADHD children decreases their risk of developing substance abuse (HAS, 2014, p. 147). This claim is supported by citing a single 2008 study in favor of this hypothesis, but cites neither the primary studies nor the 2013 meta-analysis concluding that treatment has no effect on this risk (Humphreys et al., 2013).
- *Citation distortions*: These are discrepancies in meaning between the information given in a study that has been cited and what is said by the authors citing this study. These discrepancies may result either from an alteration of the information reported by the cited study or from a truncated presentation masking a contradiction between the cited study and the conclusion drawn by the authors citing it. In the biomedical literature, approximately 10% of citations are affected by serious discrepancies that mislead the reader (Dumas-Mallet et al., 2021). I will provide an example of this below.

3.3. Media amplification of the distortions of scientific discourse

Studies in communication science have shown that the media amplify the distortions of scientific discourse when reporting on research advances. In the field of psychiatry, these studies have recently been synthesized (Dumas-Mallet & Gonon, 2020; Gonon et al., 2019). I will concentrate on the essential points here.

- *The status of initial studies and its consequences in the media*: Since they address a new issue and are generally positive, initial studies are more often published in prestigious scientific journals than subsequent studies on the same issue. They are therefore more visible to journalists. We have shown that members of the press prefer to comment on initial studies and almost never inform the public when these initial studies are contradicted by subsequent studies, which is very frequently the case (Dumas-Mallet et al., 2017). This is particularly obvious in the 1990s studies on ADHD (Gonon et al., 2012).
- *The media's emphasis on embellished results*: When embellishments are present in scientific articles, particularly in abstracts, they are most often taken up and even magnified by press releases published by scientific institutions. The media documents repeat these press releases and add a pinch of sensationalism. This phenomenon has been highlighted in several cases of media coverage of studies on ADHD (Gonon et al., 2011b).

3.4. Distortions in scientific discourse: reasons and consequences for the clinician

This brief review of the various forms of distortion in scientific discourse should in no way be taken as a disparagement of scientific research. First, it should be stressed that it is scientists themselves who regularly highlight these distortions to the public. To go back to the example given at the beginning of this section, the critical comments on the Hoogman et al. study have been made by specialists in the field. Second, researchers have an incentive to engage in these distortions: publication in prestigious journals is necessary to obtain research funding. Third, journalists have neither the time nor the expertise to investigate the scientific value of the results they report and are pressured by their editors to present them in a dramatic way. And fourth, researchers and journalists, like anyone else, are not immune to the confirmation bias that makes one prefer observations that agree with one's opinions. A thorough discussion of the reasons for and causes of these discourse distortions can be found in the four review articles cited above (Boutron & Ravaud, 2018; Dumas-Mallet & Gonon, 2020; Gonon et al., 2019; West & Bergstrom, 2021).

Many scientific articles contain a statement of the type "Our results show for the first time that...". We have seen that initial studies are often contradicted by subsequent studies. This is how the advancement of knowledge progresses. Indeed, science is a cumulative process: a promising initial study constitutes an important first step, however uncertain it may be. To become a source of knowledge, an initial study must be confirmed by other researchers. Unfortunately, the media hardly ever inform the public about the refutation of initial studies and thus contribute for years to the spread of unfounded conclusions (Bourdaa et al., 2015; Dumas-Mallet et al., 2017). Regarding the scientific argument about ADHD the print media are much more cautious than television programs (Bourdaa et al., 2015; Ponnou & Gonon, 2017). In conclusion, clinicians who wish to keep abreast of scientific advances should strive to draw their information as closely as possible from primary sources and consider initial studies with particular caution.

4. Questions

4.1. ADHD: a neurodevelopmental disorder?

If by "neurodevelopmental disorder" we simply mean that ADHD appears in childhood and involves the brain, there is no controversy: the child is a developing being and there is no behavior without a brain. Beyond that, since the group of neurodevelopmental disorders defined by DSM-V is not homogeneous from the point of view of biology or treatment, there remains the claim that these disorders are lifelong conditions (Thapar et al., 2017). Yet several epidemiological and genetic studies challenge the view that adult ADHD is necessarily a continuation of childhood ADHD (Shaw & Polanczyk, 2017).

Consequently, the term "neurodevelopmental disorder" may be accepted as a hypothesis for research, but from the practitioner's point of view, the term is not helpful. It promotes a neuro-essentialist conception of ADHD that does not encourage the clinician to look for environmental causes for the disorder such as abuse, anxiety generated by a difficult family situation or excessive exposure to screens. As has been shown for other mental disorders (Dumas-Mallet & Gonon, 2020) and neurobiological explanations of ADHD, this conception probably favors drug treatment (take for example psychostimulants, which are alleged to correct the dopamine deficit (Bourdaa et al., 2015; Gonon et al., 2011b)). Finally, if we consider the evolution of the names given to ADHD over the last two centuries, we see a fluctuation between terms evoking a brain alteration (e.g. minimal brain damage) and others that are more factual (e.g. hyperkinetic disorder). Applied to ADHD, the category "neurodevelopmental disorder" does not seem to me to be more scientifically justified than the previous neurologically based terms.

4.2. Difficulties in diagnosing ADHD

The DSM distinguishes between three types of ADHD: one in which attention deficit predominates, another in which impulsivity and hyperactivity predominate, and a third that combines the two groups of symptoms. In addition, the diagnosis of ADHD is very often associated with other disorders: anxiety, depression, bipolar disorder, behavioral and eating disorders, addictions and obesity (Faraone et al., 2021). Some researchers claim that these comorbidities do not exclude the diagnosis of ADHD and that the diagnosis is reliable despite the absence of a biological test (Faraone et al., 2021). In another article, one of these same researchers is more cautious, noting that many children diagnosed with ADHD respond as well to attention tests as children in control groups. Some children appear to show a lack of motivation for boring tasks, to perform less well in executive functions such as working memory or to experience difficulty controlling their emotions (Hinshaw, 2018). Considering such diverse symptoms and widespread comorbidities, as well as the social factors leading to the diagnosis, other researchers recommend moving forward cautiously before diagnosing ADHD and prescribing psychostimulant medication (Thomas et al., 2013). They therefore endorse what the National Institute for Health and Care Excellence (NICE, UK) has been recommending since 2013: a 10-week non-diagnostic observation period with advice for parents (Thomas et al., 2013).

4.3. Epidemic or syndemic?

In 2021, the World ADHD Federation published a consensus report signed by 82 experts in the field. They state that 5.9% of children worldwide meet the criteria for a diagnosis of ADHD, with no significant difference between countries and no change in this prevalence over the past 30 years (Faraone et al., 2021). According to this report, the increase in the diagnosis and prescription of psychostimulant drugs since 1990 is due only to a better recognition of the disorder. This report also emphasizes the high heritability rate of ADHD and the effectiveness of drug treatment (Faraone et al., 2021). These arguments encourage a neuro-essentialist conception of ADHD. It is therefore surprising to read in this report that in the USA the prevalence of ADHD is 14% in black children. In support of this very high prevalence, the researchers cite a study (Cénat et al., 2021) but fail to specify that this study attributes this prevalence to social factors (poverty, violence and the poor quality of public social and school services).

Obesity and overweight are more common in children diagnosed with ADHD (+40%), and this is even more marked in adults (+70%) (Cortese et al., 2016). A Canadian study showed that the link between obesity and ADHD in children was observed mostly in low-income families (Choudhry et al., 2013). In the USA the prescription of antipsychotics to children diagnosed with ADHD may have contributed to the correlation between ADHD and obesity. Indeed, the rapid increase of the prescribing of stimulants to children in the 1990s was followed by a sharp rise in the prescribing of antipsychotics starting in 1995 (Crystal et al., 2009). In the early 2000s, 38% of children prescribed antipsychotics had been diagnosed with ADHD even though this treatment is not recommended for this indication (Crystal et al., 2009). In the early 2010s, 22% of children diagnosed with ADHD in Texas were prescribed at least two psychotropic medications (Medhekar et al., 2019). Between 1999 and 2015 the number of US children who had been prescribed three or more psychotropic medications tripled, and of these, 85% had been diagnosed with ADHD (Zhang et al., 2021). The most common combination was a psychostimulant and an antipsychotic (Zhang et al., 2021). The prescription of antipsychotics to American children began to decline from 2008–2009 (Crystal et al., 2016) when the adverse side effects became evident: obesity, type-two diabetes, hypertension and hyperprolactinemia affect 60% of children on antipsychotics, and these effects are more severe than in adults (De Hert et al., 2011; Libowitz & Nurmi, 2021). Since prescribing antipsychotics is approximately three times as common among publicly insured (Medicaid) US children as it is among privately insured children (Crystal et al., 2016), the most disadvantaged children have been, and still are, the most exposed to these iatrogenic effects, albeit to a lesser extent more recently (Zito et al., 2018).

Within a given country, income disparities between the richest and poorest people lead to adverse consequences for families (such as run-down neighborhoods, poor-quality public schools and social services, violent environments and poor nutrition) that increase the risk of ADHD, obesity and chronic cardio-metabolic diseases (Pickett & Wilkinson, 2015). I further hypothesize that the prescription of psychostimulants to ADHD children opens the door to the prescription of antipsychotics, and this suggests an iatrogenic influence contributing to the correlation between ADHD and obesity. In this context, I find the concept of syndemics interesting. Its proponents argue for a less compartmentalized view of health (Mendenhall et al., 2017; Singer et al., 2017). They highlight the interactions between chronic pathologies as well as their social determinants. These interactions have been further expanded with COVID-19 as the mortality rate due to the virus is significantly increased in people with obesity and chronic cardio-metabolic diseases (Mendenhall, 2020).

5.   Conclusion

Part of the scientific discourse encourages a narrow biomedical and neuro-essentialist conception of ADHD. However, this conception is not effective when it comes to helping struggling children and parents. It minimizes the social context, especially where prevention could be effective (e.g. exposure to screens or premature birth). It fails to take full account of health and education issues, including iatrogenic effects.

Along with many others, I advocate taking into account the psychological and social context when practitioners undertake to help children and their parents. More than a neuroscientific justification, what they need is to be heard in their complexity and specificity. In terms of population, perhaps we need to think further. One major fact remains unexplained: the prevalence of ADHD is two to three times higher in boys than in girls. Consistent with this difference, the gap in academic success in all developed countries is widening in favor of girls. Marcel Gauchet attributes this difference to the major cultural changes that took place in the 1970s: the end of male domination made it more difficult for boys to construct their sexual identity, whereas it made it easier for girls. According to Gauchet, this cultural upheaval contributed to many boys' academic apathy (Gauchet, 2018).

The term ADHD covers an extremely wide range of difficulties. Understanding them no doubt requires less neuroscience and more human and social sciences.

References

Batstra, L., Te Meerman, S., Conners, K., & Frances, A. (2017). Subcortical brain volume differences in participants with attention deficit hyperactivity disorder in children and adults. *Lancet Psychiatry*, *4*(6), 439.

Baweja, R., Mattison, R. E., & Waxmonsky, J. G. (2015). Impact of attention-deficit hyperactivity disorder on school performance: What are the effects of medication? *Paediatric Drugs*, *17*(6), 459–477.

Bodkin, H. (2017, February 16). ADHD is a brain disorder, not a label for poor parenting, say scientists. *The Telegraph*. https://www.telegraph.co.uk/science/2017/02/15/adhd -brain-disorder-not-label-poor-parenting-say-scientists/

Bourdaa, M., Konsman, J. P., Secail, C., Venturini, T., Veyrat-Masson, I., & Gonon, F. (2015). Does television reflect the evolution of scientific knowledge? The case of attention deficit hyperactivity disorder coverage on French TV. *Public Understanding of Science*, *24*(2), 200–209.

Boutron, I., & Ravaud, P. (2018). Misrepresentation and distortion of research in biomedical literature. *Proceedings of the National Academy of Sciences USA*, *115*(11), 2613–2619.

Campbell, S. B., Douglas, V. I., & Morgenstern, G. (1971). Cognitive styles in hyperactive children and the effect of methylphenidate. *The Journal of Child Psychology and Psychiatry*, *12*(1), 55–67.

Cénat, J. M., Blais-Rochette, C., Morse, C., Vandette, M. P., Noorishad, P. G., Kogan, C., … Labelle, P. R. (2021). Prevalence and risk factors associated with attention-deficit/ hyperactivity disorder among US black individuals: A systematic review and meta- analysis. *JAMA Psychiatry*, *78*(1), 21–28.

Choudhry, Z., Sengupta, S. M., Grizenko, N., Harvey, W. J., Fortier, M., Schmitz, N., & Joober, R. (2013). Body weight and ADHD: Examining the role of self-regulation. *PLoS One*, *8*(1), e55351.

Cortese, S., Aoki, Y. Y., Itahashi, T., Castellanos, F. X., & Eickhoff, S. B. (2021). Systematic review and meta-analysis: Resting-state functional magnetic resonance imaging studies of attention-deficit/hyperactivity disorder. *Journal of the American Academy of Child & Adolescent Psychiatry*, *60*(1), 61–75.

Cortese, S., Moreira-Maia, C. R., St Fleur, D., Morcillo-Peñalver, C., Rohde, L. A., & Faraone, S. V. (2016). Association between ADHD and obesity: A systematic review and meta-analysis. *The American Journal of Psychiatry*, *173*(1), 34–43.

Crystal, S., Mackie, T., Fenton, M. C., Amin, S., Neese-Todd, S., Olfson, M., & Bilder, S. (2016). Rapid growth of antipsychotic prescriptions for children who are publicly insured has ceased, but concerns remain. *Health Affairs (Millwood)*, *35*(6), 974–982.

Crystal, S., Olfson, M., Huang, C., Pincus, H., & Gerhard, T. (2009). Broadened use of atypical antipsychotics: Safety, effectiveness, and policy challenges. *Health Affairs (Millwood)*, *28*(5), 770–781.

De Hert, M., Dobbelaere, M., Sheridan, E. M., Cohen, D., & Correll, C. U. (2011). Metabolic and endocrine adverse effects of second-generation antipsychotics in children and adolescents: A systematic review of randomized, placebo controlled trials and guidelines for clinical practice. *European Psychiatry*, *26*(3), 144–158.

Dumas-Mallet, E., Boraud, T., & Gonon, F. (2021). Le mésusage des citations et ses conséquences en médecine. *Médecine/Sciences (Paris)*, *37*(11), 1035–1041.

Dumas-Mallet, E., Button, K., Boraud, T., Munafo, M., & Gonon, F. (2016). Replication validity of initial association studies: A comparison between psychiatry, neurology and four somatic diseases. *PLoS One*, *11*(6), e0158064.

Dumas-Mallet, E., & Gonon, F. (2020). Messaging in biological psychiatry: Misrepresentations, their causes, and potential consequences. *Harvard Review of Psychiatry*, *28*(6), 395–403.

Dumas-Mallet, E., Smith, A., Boraud, T., & Gonon, F. (2017). Poor replication validity of biomedical association studies reported by newspapers. *PLoS One*, *12*(2), e0172650.

Faraone, S. V., Banaschewski, T., Coghill, D., Zheng, Y., Biederman, J., Bellgrove, M. A., … Wang, Y. (2021). The World Federation of ADHD International Consensus Statement: 208 evidence-based conclusions about the disorder. *Neuroscience & Biobehavioral Reviews*, *128*, 789–818.

Fulton, B. D., Scheffler, R. M., & Hinshaw, S. P. (2015). State variation in increased ADHD prevalence: Links to NCLB school accountability and state medication laws. *Psychiatric Services*, *66*(10), 1074–1082.

Galera, C., Cote, S. M., Bouvard, M. P., Pingault, J. B., Melchior, M., Michel, G., … Tremblay, R. E. (2011). Early risk factors for hyperactivity-impulsivity and inattention trajectories from age 17 months to 8 years. *Archives of General Psychiatry*, *68*(12), 1267–1275.

Gauchet, M. (2018). La fin de la domination masculine. *Le Débat*, *200*, 75–98.

Goldenberg, R. L., Culhane, J. F., Iams, J. D., & Romero, R. (2008). Epidemiology and causes of preterm birth. *Lancet*, *371*(9606), 75–84.

Gonon, F., Bezard, E., & Boraud, T. (2011a). What should be said to the lay public regarding ADHD etiology. *American Journal of Medical Genetics Part B: Neuropsychiatric Genetics*, *156*(8), 989–991.

Gonon, F., Bézard, E., & Boraud, T. (2011b). Misrepresentation of neuroscience data might give rise to misleading conclusions in the media: The case of attention deficit hyperactivity disorder. *PLoS One*, *6*(1), e14618.

Gonon, F., & Cohen, D. (2011). Le trouble déficitaire de l'attention avec hyperactivité: la génétique est-elle impliquée? *Médecine/Sciences (Paris)*, *27*(3), 315–317.

Gonon, F., Dumas-Mallet, E., & Ponnou, S. (2019). La couverture médiatique des observations scientifiques concernant les troubles mentaux. *Les Cahiers du journalisme*, *2*(3), R45–R63.

Gonon, F., Konsman, J. P., Cohen, D., & Boraud, T. (2012). Why most biomedical findings echoed by newspapers turn out to be false: The case of Attention Deficit Hyperactivity Disorder. *PLoS One*, *7*(9), e44275.

Haute Autorité de Santé (HAS). (2014). Conduite à tenir en médecine de premier recours devant un enfant ou un adolescent susceptible d'avoir un trouble déficit de l'attention avec ou sans hyperactivité. https://www.has-sante.fr/jcms/c_1362146/fr/conduite-a-tenir-en-medecine-de-premier-recours-devant-un-enfant-ou-un-adolescent-susceptible-d-avoir-un-trouble-deficit-de-l-attention-avec-ou-sans-hyperactivite

Hinshaw, S. P. (2018). Attention Deficit Hyperactivity Disorder (ADHD): Controversy, developmental mechanisms, and multiple levels of analysis. *Annual Review of Clinical Psychology*, *14*, 291–316.

Hoogman, M., Bralten, J., Hibar, D. P., Mennes, M., Zwiers, M. P., Schweren, L. S. J., … Franke, B. (2017). Subcortical brain volume differences in participants with attention deficit hyperactivity disorder in children and adults: A cross-sectional mega-analysis. *Lancet Psychiatry, 4*(4), 310–319.

Hoogman, M., Buitelaar, J. K., Faraone, S. V., Shaw, P., & Franke, B. (2017). Subcortical brain volume differences in participants with attention deficit hyperactivity disorder in children and adults – authors' reply. *Lancet Psychiatry, 4*(6), 440–441.

Humphreys, K. L., Eng, T., & Lee, S. S. (2013). Stimulant medication and substance use outcomes: A meta-analysis. *JAMA Psychiatry, 70*(7), 740–749.

Jangmo, A., Stålhandske, A., Chang, Z., Chen, Q., Almqvist, C., Feldman, I., ... Larsson, H. (2019). Attention-deficit/hyperactivity disorder, school performance, and effect of medication. *Journal of the American Academy of Child & Adolescent Psychiatry, 58*(4), 423–432.

Lange, K. W., Reichl, S., Lange, K. M., Tucha, L., & Tucha, O. (2010). The history of attention deficit hyperactivity disorder. *ADHD Attention Deficit and Hyperactivity Disorders, 2*(4), 241–255.

Libowitz, M. R., & Nurmi, E. L. (2021). The burden of antipsychotic-induced weight gain and metabolic syndrome in children. *Frontiers in Psychiatry, 12*, 623681.

Mahone, E. M., & Denckla, M. B. (2017). Attention-deficit/hyperactivity disorder: A historical neuropsychological perspective. *Journal of the International Neuropsychological Society, 23*(9–10), 916–929.

Martinez-Badía, J., & Martinez-Raga, J. (2015). Who says this is a modern disorder? The early history of attention deficit hyperactivity disorder. *World Journal of Psychiatry, 5*(4), 379–386.

Mayes, R., Bagwell, C., & Erkulwater, J. (2008). ADHD and the rise in stimulant use among children. *Harvard Review of Psychiatry, 16*(3), 151–166.

Medhekar, R., Aparasu, R., Bhatara, V., Johnson, M., Alonzo, J., Schwarzwald, H., & Chen, H. (2019). Risk factors of psychotropic polypharmacy in the treatment of children and adolescents with psychiatric disorders. *Research in Social and Administrative Pharmacy, 15*(4), 395–403.

Mendenhall, E. (2020). The COVID-19 syndemic is not global: Context matters. *Lancet, 396*(10264), 1731.

Mendenhall, E., Kohrt, B. A., Norris, S. A., Ndetei, D., & Prabhakaran, D. (2017). Non-communicable disease syndemics: Poverty, depression, and diabetes among low-income populations. *Lancet, 389*(10072), 951–963.

Pickett, K. E., & Wilkinson, R. G. (2015). Income inequality and health: A causal review. *Social Science & Medicine, 128*, 316–326.

Ponnou, S., & Gonon, F. (2017). How French media have portrayed ADHD to the lay public and to social workers. *International Journal of Qualitative Studies on Health and Well-being, 12*(Sup1), 1298244.

Prasad, V., Brogan, E., Mulvaney, C., Grainge, M., Stanton, W., & Sayal, K. (2013). How effective are drug treatments for children with ADHD at improving on-task behaviour and academic achievement in the school classroom? A systematic review and meta-analysis. *European Child & Adolescent Psychiatry, 22*(4), 203–216.

Raman, S. R., Man, K. K. C., Bahmanyar, S., Berard, A., Bilder, S., Boukhris, T., ... Wong, I. C. K. (2018). Trends in attention-deficit hyperactivity disorder medication use: A retrospective observational study using population-based databases. *Lancet Psychiatry, 5*(10), 824–835.

Samea, F., Soluki, S., Nejati, V., Zarei, M., Cortese, S., Eickhoff, S. B., … Eickhoff, C. R. (2019). Brain alterations in children/adolescents with ADHD revisited: A neuroimaging meta-analysis of 96 structural and functional studies. *Neuroscience & Biobehavioral Reviews*, *100*, 1–8.

Sharpe, K. (2014). Medication: The smart-pill oversell. *Nature*, *506*(7487), 146–148.

Shaw, P., & Polanczyk, G. V. (2017). Combining epidemiological and neurobiological perspectives to characterize the lifetime trajectories of ADHD. *European Child & Adolescent Psychiatry*, *26*(2), 139–141.

Singer, M., Bulled, N., Ostrach, B., & Mendenhall, E. (2017). Syndemics and the biosocial conception of health. *Lancet*, *389*(10072), 941–950.

Smith, M. (2017). Hyperactive around the world? The history of ADHD in global perspective. *Social History of Medicine*, *30*(4), 767–787.

Tamana, S. K., Ezeugwu, V., Chikuma, J., Lefebvre, D. L., Azad, M. B., Moraes, T. J., … Mandhane, P. J. (2019). Screen-time is associated with inattention problems in preschoolers: Results from the CHILD birth cohort study. *PLoS One*, *14*(4), e0213995.

Thapar, A. (2018). Discoveries on the genetics of ADHD in the 21st century: New findings and their implications. *The American Journal of Psychiatry*, *175*(10), 943–950.

Thapar, A., & Cooper, M. (2016). Attention deficit hyperactivity disorder. *Lancet*, *387*(10024), 1240–1250.

Thapar, A., Cooper, M., & Rutter, M. (2017). Neurodevelopmental disorders. *Lancet Psychiatry*, *4*(4), 339–346.

The MTA Cooperative Group. (1999). A 14-month randomized clinical trial of treatment strategies for attention-deficit/hyperactivity disorder. *Archives of General Psychiatry*, *56*(12), 1073–1086.

Thomas, R., Mitchell, G. K., & Batstra, L. (2013). Attention-deficit/hyperactivity disorder: Are we helping or harming? *BMJ*, *347*, f6172.

Visser, S. N., Danielson, M. L., Bitsko, R. H., Holbrook, J. R., Kogan, M. D., Ghandour, R. M., … Blumberg, S. J. (2014). Trends in the parent-report of health care provider-diagnosed and medicated attention-deficit/hyperactivity disorder: United States, 2003–2011. *Journal of the American Academy of Child & Adolescent Psychiatry*, *53*(1), 34–46.e32.

Weiss, M. D., Baer, S., Allan, B. A., Saran, K., & Schibuk, H. (2011). The screens culture: Impact on ADHD. *ADHD Attention Deficit and Hyperactivity Disorders*, *3*(4), 327–334.

West, J. D., & Bergstrom, C. T. (2021). Misinformation in and about science. *Proceedings of the National Academy of Sciences USA*, *118*(15), e1912444117.

Whitely, M., Raven, M., Timimi, S., Jureidini, J., Phillimore, J., Leo, J., … Landman, P. (2019). Annual Research Review: Attention deficit hyperactivity disorder late birthdate effect common in both high and low prescribing international jurisdictions: A systematic review. *The Journal of Child Psychology and Psychiatry*, *60*(4), 380–391.

Wolraich, M. L., Chan, E., Froehlich, T., Lynch, R. L., Bax, A., Redwine, S. T., … Hagan, J. F., Jr. (2019). ADHD diagnosis and treatment guidelines: A historical perspective. *Pediatrics*, *144*(4), e20191682.

Zhang, C., Spence, O., Reeves, G., & dosReis, S. (2021). Characteristics of youths treated with psychotropic polypharmacy in the United States, 1999 to 2015. *JAMA Pediatrics*, *175*(2), 196–198.

Zito, J. M., Burcu, M., McKean, S., Warnock, R., & Kelman, J. (2018). Pediatric use of antipsychotic medications before and after Medicaid peer review implementation. *JAMA Psychiatry*, *75*(1), 100–103.

Chapter 2

Listening to children rather than to the sirens of scientism

Patrick Landman

***

1. Introduction

The diagnosis of ADD/ADHD will long continue to be the subject of criticism, contestation and controversy, all of which began as soon as this diagnosis first appeared in the complex and shifting sphere of psychiatric nosography.

Its undeniable "success" – it is on the way to becoming the most common reason for consultation in child psychiatry – can in no way serve as scientific validation. It is rather the consequence of various combined factors:

- The evolution of the demand in child psychiatry focusing on the sedation of behavioral symptoms;
- The importance given to academic performance as a result of selection and the legitimate concern of parents;
- The tendency to deny pedagogical, educational and social problems by replacing them with alleged brain-related troubles;
- Big Pharma's propaganda relayed by family associations and two other factors that I will insist on: *scientism in psychiatry* and *the tendency to deny psychological suffering.*

So why is this diagnosis a favorite target for criticism by professionals? There are many reasons for this, and they have been outlined in a number of studies. In my opinion, the main reason is that ADD/ADHD is a typical example of the successful invasion by scientism of current mainstream psychiatric paradigms.

2. The temptation of scientism

The term "scientism" has indeed become pejorative, but this was not necessarily the case a century ago in Freud's day. It could at that time refer to a bias in favor of scientific rationality whose epistemological value for access to knowledge was

DOI: 10.4324/9781003584469-3

considered superior to all other approaches – especially philosophical or religious. Scientism can be defined as follows:

> Scientism is a position that emerged in the 19th century, according to which experimental science is the only reliable source of knowledge about the world, as opposed to religious revelations, superstitions, traditions, customs and all other forms of knowledge. Scientism therefore proposed, in the words of Ernest Renan, 'to organize humanity scientifically'. It was therefore a matter of trust or a wager (or a hope). The term *faith* does not apply, in principle, to the application of the principles and methods of science, including modern science, in all fields. The core of this position can be summarized as follows: 'Science (truly) describes the world as it is'.
>
> (https://fr.m.wikipedia.org/wiki/Scientisme)

It is obvious that the ambition of the promoters of DSM-III and subsequent versions was to organize psychiatry scientifically. However, 40 years after DSM-III, psychiatry has remained in the prescientific era. Knowledge in psychiatry is made up of the coexistence of forms of knowledge of different ages that are difficult to compare because their epistemological orientation and mode of production are too dissimilar.

Moreover, no classification can be considered absolutely superior to others. The DSM is the object of a certain broad consensus, but this fact results from the choices made in the production of the DSM (to privilege observable behaviors, or to refuse any theoretical a priori, for instance). This is not related to any scientific validity. In fact, psychiatric clinical practice is at the intersection of several different domains: 1) a medical semiological domain, useful for prescribing medication, for example; 2) a domain that could be described as systemic or sociological, which takes into account family, environmental and cultural dimensions; and finally 3) an intra-psychological domain, which concerns the psychological functioning of the subject suffering from a pathology and the meanings they give to their symptoms and suffering. The result of this complexity is that no classification can satisfactorily guide good psychiatric practice. Although the recommendations based on these classifications can be useful as an aid to decision-making, they can in no way represent injunctions that can be enforced on practitioners.

The "success" of ADD/ADHD is based on the prestige of medical science, which mainly rests on modern research and the faith it generates in public opinion, in political decision-makers and in the senior health administration.

Research is traditionally divided into basic research on the one hand and applied research on the other. This division is criticized by some authors, but it seems useful to me in my discussion of ADHD. Whereas basic research seeks to identify one or more natural laws and their consequences (such as a causal agent, or simply the biological markers of a disease), applied research depends on "doing": the relevance of its results is measured by criteria of effectiveness.

3. Disappointing results in the diagnosis of ADD/ADHD in both kinds of research

3.1. The search for biological causes and markers

To the question *What is ADD/ADHD?*, websites or articles for the general public yield a variety of answers. Here is a non-exhaustive but representative selection:

"ADD/ADHD stands for Attention Deficit/Hyperactivity Disorder. It is a medical condition. A person with ADHD has differences in brain development and activity that affect attention, the capacity to sit still, and self-control. ADD/ADHD can affect the child at school, at home and in his relationships with friends."

"If you have Attention Deficit Hyperactivity Disorder (ADHD), you may have a lot of energy and find it hard to concentrate. It can be hard to control your speech and actions. ADD/ADHD is the most common behavioral disorder in children. It usually starts around 18 months of age, but symptoms become noticeable between 3 and 7 years of age. We don't know what causes ADHD, but experts think it is hereditary. It may also be caused by an imbalance of brain chemicals."

"ADD/ADHD is characterized by periods of impulsivity, hyperactivity and inattention, but it involves much more than being a dreamer or a joker. ADHD affects between 2 and 5% of the population and is largely genetic, although environmental factors can make it worse."

It is clear from these quotes that ADD/ADHD is presented to the general public as an undeniable pathology, a natural entity of biological – probably genetic – origin, insufficiently diagnosed and curable by medication. All these statements are questionable and even misleading. We will examine them in the following section.

3.2. ADD/ADHD: an undeniable pathology?

Like any psychiatric diagnosis, ADHD is descriptive, not explanatory. It cannot be compared to a medical diagnosis such as tuberculosis caused by a bacillus or diabetes resulting from a blood sugar dysfunction. Imagine saying to a parent, "Your child has attentional difficulties as evidenced by a neuropsychological test (he has impulsive behaviors, etc.), so he has ADD/ADHD." Now, if this parent asks you: "Why does he have ADD/ADHD?", the only relevant answer in the current state of knowledge will be: "Because he has attentional difficulties and impulsive behaviors." In other words, what we are dealing with here is a tautological line of reasoning, not an explanation.

What then is the basis for ADD/ADHD proponents to "prove" the existence of this disorder? We will now take a look at some of the supposed "scientific evidence for ADD/ADHD".

3.3. Genetic evidence

The claim that ADHD is genetic[1] has been extrapolated from studying twins. In the twin-study method, it is assumed that when a higher percentage of identical twins than fraternal twins are diagnosed with the same disorder, it is due to genetic rather than environmental factors. This is because identical twin pairs share 100% of their genetic makeup, whereas fraternal twins share an average of 50% of their genes. However, in order for identical twins to have a greater likelihood of suffering from a disorder because they share the same genes, it must be assumed that the psychosocial environment is the same for both identical and fraternal twins. This is called the environmental equality hypothesis. It has long been established that this hypothesis does not hold when comparing identical and fraternal twins. Identical twins are often treated similarly (e.g., they wear the same clothes) and experience a unique psychological environment (e.g., they swap roles to confuse others). Being an identical twin is a different experience from being a fraternal twin, and the psychosocial environment alone (in addition to genes) could therefore be responsible for greater behavioral or emotional similarity between identical than between fraternal twins. This means that the twin-study method does not distinguish between genetic and environmental factors for "psychiatric" cases and that this method does not measure the genetic contribution to ADHD.

The only way to reliably identify a specific genetic contribution to ADHD is through molecular genetic studies. Since faster and cheaper whole-genome scans have become available, molecular genetic evidence has mounted. This growing body of research into the genetics of ADHD has not revealed any particular genetic findings, either abnormal genes or consistent genetic associations. Yet this has not stopped unscrupulous researchers from claiming otherwise.

A 2010 study published in *The Lancet* claimed to have found concrete molecular genetic evidence that ADHD is genetic (Williams et al., 2010). This study was, and continues to be, referenced as the preeminent study demonstrating that ADHD can be considered a genetic disorder with absolute certainty. In the press release issued at the time, the head of the research team, Professor Anita Thapar, left little room for doubt when she announced, "We can now say with certainty that ADHD is a genetic disorder and that the brains of children with this disorder develop differently from those of other children." Here is what they actually found: the study compared whole-genome scans of 366 children "with ADHD" with those of 1,047 control children "without ADHD", looking for what are called copy number variants (CNVs). CNVs are abnormal pieces of genetic code that are repeated or deleted where they should not be. The researchers found that 15.5% (57) of the children with ADHD had CNVs compared to 7.5% (78) of the control children without ADHD. This leaves an excess of 8% in the ADHD group, a figure that is hardly significant. If we are to accept the standard prevalence quoted by the mainstream view of ADHD, it also means that if you meet a young person with CNVs, he or she is more likely to be undiagnosed as having ADHD than diagnosed as having the disorder.

But the deception does not end there. The average recorded IQ of children with ADHD was 86, i.e., 14 points lower than the general population average of 100. Furthermore, when 33 ADHD children with intellectual disabilities (IQ below 70) were excluded from the ADHD group, only 11.4% of the remaining 333 children had CNVs (only 4% more than the non-ADHD control group). Of the 33 children with ADHD and intellectual disabilities, 39% (13) had CNVs. These data are more suggestive of a relationship between the presence of CNVs and intellectual disability (39%) than of one between the presence of CNVs and ADHD (11.4%). The authors of this study should have controlled for IQ given its disproportionate impact on CNV levels, but they chose not to. As mentioned above, the average IQ in the ADHD group was significantly lower than that of the control group (whose population average IQ can be assumed to be 100). The authors should have chosen a subgroup of their ADHD patients who had an average IQ of 100. This would have provided a more legitimate comparison group with their control group. One cannot help but wonder if this choice had not in fact been made, as it can be supposed that the researchers may have ended up with a zero difference or negligible difference of about 1% and therefore chosen not to make it public.

This type of high-profile, media attention–grabbing publication is worse than junk science: the authors have misled the medical community and the general public in their conclusions. As far as genetics is concerned, no evidence was found, so the null hypothesis can thus be maintained: there is no identifiable abnormality or characteristic genetic profile associated with ADHD.

3.4. Has brain imaging, which is regarded as the microscope of the 21st century, allowed us to identify markers?

As with genetics, brain imaging studies of ADHD have not shown any specific or characteristic abnormality. The picture that emerges is one of consistently inconsistent results from studies of small samples, not always homogeneous with respect to the children's age. This is an important factor, one I will comment on below. These studies generally do not control for IQ levels or possible drug effects. The results show only statistical discrepancies: the children's brains do not seem to be recognized by radiologists as clinically abnormal. One research team finds that one part of the brain is smaller than that of the "healthy" control group, and another team does not, or even finds that this same part is slightly larger.

But, as I mentioned before, why should science get in the way of a fervent scientist? In 2017, *The Lancet Psychiatry* published a study that, according to the authors, provided definitive proof that young people with ADHD have different and smaller brains than their healthy peers (Hoogman et al., 2017). As with the junk science surrounding genetics, lead researcher Dr. Hoogman's bold claims do not stand up to scrutiny. In a press release covered by the mainstream media, he said, "The results of our study confirm that people with ADHD have differences in their brain structure and thus suggest that ADHD is a brain disorder." In an excellent analysis for *Mad in America*, Michael Corrigan and Robert Whitaker show how the research reveals more about the authors' desperation to find something than their ability to conduct a scientifically careful analysis of their results (Corrigan & Whitaker, 2017).

The authors call their study a "mega-analysis" because they took data from a large number of previous research projects and "crunched" the results from different sites around the world as if it were one big study. This process is sometimes illuminating, but it can also make incidental results seem more important than they are. In total, they had data from the brain scans of 1,713 patients diagnosed with ADHD and of 1,529 people not diagnosed, collected from 23 different sites globally. They say that what amounts to negligible differences in particular brain structures (not all of them) becomes statistically significant when they add up all the recorded volumes available for a particular structure in the ADHD and non-ADHD groups. The use of some measures of statistical variance allows them to claim that the differences are so small that they have no clinical relevance. This method allows them to hide consistently inconsistent results.

For example, the largest difference was found for a tiny brain structure called the nucleus accumbens (NAc). This mega-analysis says that children with ADHD have a smaller NAc. However, if you look at the data by geographical site, you find ten sites that found a smaller NAc on average in the ADHD group, four sites that found a larger NAc in the ADHD group, and six sites that found no difference. These results concern the brain structure that presents the greatest difference according to the study. There are other major technical problems with the interpretation of the NAc scans. For example, people in Bergen, Norway have an average NAc volume of 758 mm^3 vs. 805 mm^3 (ADHD vs. control group), whereas in Würzburg, Germany they have an average NAc volume of 462 mm^3 vs. 449 mm^3 (ADHD vs. control group). Norwegian children may have surprisingly high NAcs compared to German children, who by this standard would all have severe ADHD. Note, however, that it is the Norwegian control group that has larger volumes, while the German ADHD group has larger volumes. Given this huge variation – which is greater between centers than within a center – there is a further bias in the results: those with the largest total volumes are found in the population whose control group had larger NAcs.

This is yet another study that does not take into account differences in IQ. Associations between brain size and IQ have been found in a whole series of studies of adults and children. When the authors of this study published the correct IQ table (embarrassingly, they had originally published an incorrect version), a separate group re-analyzed their data, controlling for potential IQ effects, and concluded that there was no significant difference between people with ADHD and the control group in any of the brain areas studied when the IQ difference was controlled.

Again, there is no conclusive scientific evidence. No one has been able to find a characteristic abnormality and, therefore, there is no biological marker or brain scan used to diagnose ADHD. The null hypothesis stands: there is no characteristic brain abnormality associated with ADHD.

3.5. Sami Timimi and the application of the famous "chemical imbalance" theory to ADHD

As Sami Timimi argues,[2] there is no shortage of "experts" willing to assert that ADHD is related to a lack or chemical imbalance of the dopamine neurotransmitters. This idea is based solely on the fact that drugs (such as Ritalin®) that act to stimulate the release of dopamine and therefore increase its levels in the brain's synapses seem to improve the "symptoms" of ADHD. Decades ago, studies showed that taking stimulants, regardless of the diagnosis, improves the ability to stay focused on a task, at least in the short term. However, since no one had yet demonstrated the absence or lack of dopamine in people diagnosed with ADHD, the chemical imbalance theory was allowed to spread, along with aggressive marketing on the part of those drug manufacturers whose products increase the levels of these chemicals in the brain.

Every so often, a study that challenges conventional wisdom gets some attention, albeit limited. One such study was published in 2013 (del Campo et al., 2013). Its findings challenge previous conclusions that ADHD results from fundamental irregularities in dopamine transmission. The researchers found that administering methylphenidate (better known as Ritalin®) to healthy adult volunteers as well as those with ADHD symptoms led to similar increases in the brain chemical dopamine. Both groups also showed equivalent levels of improvement from the drug when tested on their ability to concentrate and pay attention.

The null hypothesis is once again maintained: there is no characteristic chemical imbalance associated with ADHD.

3.6. Immaturity or age gap as confounding factors

Several studies conducted in different countries have found that the youngest children in their class – for example, children born in December – have a significantly higher risk of being diagnosed with ADHD than older children born in January. These studies have shown that this pattern is recurrent, be it in countries with high rates of diagnosis or prescription (such as the United States) or with low rates (such as Finland). Such a pattern of ADHD identification and diagnosis strongly suggests that relative immaturity compared to one's peers is a significant risk factor for receiving this label (i.e., for adults noting and problematizing the described behaviors associated with ADHD). Whether more than 6% of children (in the Icelandic study) are prescribed stimulants or less than 1% (in the Finnish study), the pattern remains the same. Whatever cultural norms are used to problematize these behaviors, relative immaturity within the class always appears to be a risk factor. Of course, children mature at different rates, which raises the important question of whether a diagnosis of ADHD, even for the oldest children in the class, might also reflect their relatively slower development.

For some time, I have believed that the increase in pseudo-diagnoses such as ADHD is a reflection of the growing intolerance of diversity in children. From an early age, children are given messages that they are valued and appreciated for what they do (for their "performance", especially in school) rather than for who they are. These findings reinforce the concern that the prevalence of diagnoses such as ADHD acts as a barometer of our intolerance of children and of their immature behaviors that sometimes trouble us more than they trouble them.

4.   The denial of psychological suffering and the limits of ADHD for the clinical practice

The refusal to acknowledge the psychological suffering of children leads many parents to reject any approach through the psyche and even to deny the very existence of the psyche. These parents, for understandable reasons, prefer to favor theories that only take into account the approach that puts forward alleged brain-related abnormalities. Assuming that such abnormalities exist and that we manage to prove their existence, thus eliminating any psychological causality, this will not erase the question of the psyche given that a recognized organic disease can lead to serious psychological disorders: a human subject suffering from such a disease may feel the need to talk about it. When I was a psychiatrist in training, I had the feeling that I was learning a sort of brainless psychiatry, which was understandable because of the lack of scientific progress in the field of brain functioning. Nowadays, with the advances in imaging and neuroscience, we learn psychiatry without a psyche, which is just as regrettable.

I will end with a short clinical observation that illustrates the value of listening to children labeled ADD/ADHD and of taking into account their psychological suffering.

Years ago, I saw in my office a 12-year-old child I will call André. André had been diagnosed with ADHD and treated with methylphenidate for several years with limited success. His parents felt that the treatment was no longer serving its purpose but wanted advice because they felt that the prescription was being renewed too automatically. The boy, however, did not want to stop the medication, which he thought protected him.

Ever since the child had begun treatment, he had been tested, diagnosed and medicated, but never asked to speak except to answer the ritual questions dictated by protocol. I decided to continue the prescription, but also to see this child more often than the simple prescription renewal required. This way of proceeding was suggested to me by Jean Chambry. The time lag between the frequency of the interviews and the frequency of the methylphenidate prescription renewal makes it possible to first establish a strong therapeutic complicity, then to present oneself, thanks to this time lag, as someone other than a prescriber who submits to the scheduled renewal of prescriptions. This may lead to a space for discussion favoring transference.

After a few appointments, André agreed to talk. He told me that he was unhappy because his parents did not get along, that they often quarreled and that he could hear them because his room was only separated from his parents' room by a partition. He told me that he felt guilty, that he thought he was responsible for these quarrels because of his behavioral problems, and that this was why he was afraid to stop the medication.

I saw the parents with their son. They were very emphatic about the need for André to have a good education and to do well in school, and as they spoke André became very agitated. Then I asked the parents if their own "good education" had been an asset in their lives, and the father explained at length that his education had done him little good and that he had succeeded in life thanks to other qualities. I watched as André listened to his father's candid admission and gradually calmed down.

Several weeks later, the mother asked to see me alone without her husband and son. She was in tears: her husband had decided to separate from her to live with a man.

They had not been intimate for a long time, her husband using fatigue and weight gain as reasons for his lack of desire. But that her husband might be homosexual had never crossed her mind. She asked me to continue talking to André and to provide her with a reference.

Without going any further with this story, I would like to offer some thoughts. The behavioral diagnosis of ADHD with a long-term prescription had taken center stage. It had made it possible to conceal the fragility of the parents' relationship, the father's half-lies, the concealment of his homosexuality, the mother's depression and above all the child's psychological suffering. André used medication to try to alleviate this psychological suffering. Listening to what André had to say had helped to unravel his situation a little. It was probably important that I not stop the prescription at first, since this created in André a feeling of confidence. The clinic of listening and the transferential clinic can only proceed case by case; it excludes protocol and any ideological or dogmatic posture.

Methylphenidate is a medication that works in the short term in many cases. It improves attention, especially for tedious tasks. It generally has few side effects, but these can be serious, such as an impact on growth or anorexia. Its long-term effects are poorly documented, and it stabilizes a child's development only if prescribing it is accompanied by support and by psychological or even social guidance. In the absence of this support, it becomes a performance-enhancing drug that can long mask underlying pathologies hidden by the superficial diagnosis of ADD/ADHD. It is by no means a magic pill.

Notes

1 https://www.madinamerica.com/2020/11/insane-medicine-chapter-3-part-1/
2 Sami Timimi is a psychiatrist and professor at Lincoln University in England.

Bibliography

American Psychiatric Association (APA). (1966). *Diagnostic Statistical Manual of Mental Disorders, Second Edition (DSM-2)*. Washington, DC: APA.

American Psychiatric Association (APA). (1980). *Diagnostic Statistical Manual of Mental Disorders, Third Edition (DSM-3)*. Washington, DC: APA.

American Psychiatric Association (APA). (1987). *Diagnostic and Statistical Manual of Mental Disorders, Third Edition Revised (DSM-3-R)*. Washington, DC: APA.

American Psychiatric Association (APA). (1994). *Diagnostic and Statistical Manual of Mental Disorders, Fourth Edition (DSM-4)*. Washington, DC: APA.

American Psychiatric Association (APA). (2013). *Diagnostic and Statistical Manual of Mental Disorders, Fifth Edition (DSM-5)*. Washington, DC: APA.

Bejerot, S., Nilsonne, G., & Humble, M. B. (2017). Subcortical brain volume differences in participants with attention deficit hyperactivity disorder in children and adults. *Lancet Psychiatry*, *4*(6), 437.

Bradley, C. (1937). The behaviour of children receiving Benzedrine. *American Journal of Psychiatry*, *94*(3), 577–585.

Brewis, A., & Schmidt, K. (2003). Gender variation in the identification of Mexican children's psychiatric symptoms. *Medical Anthropology Quarterly*, *17*(3), 376–393.

Carpenter-Song, E. (2008). Caught in the psychiatric net: Meanings and experiences of ADHD, pediatric bipolar disorder and mental health treatment among a diverse group of families in the United States. *Culture, Medicine, and Psychiatry*, *33*(1), 61–85.

Conrad, P. (1975). The discovery of hyperkinesis: Notes on the medicalization of deviant behavior. *Social Problems*, *23*(1), 12–21.

Corrigan, M. W., & Whitaker, R. (2017, April 15). Lancet Psychiatry needs to retract the ADHD-enigma study. *Mad in America*. https://www.madinamerica.com/2017/04/lancet -psychiatry-needs-to-retract-the-adhd-enigma-study/

Curtin, K., Fleckenstein, A. E., Keeshin, B. R., Yurgelun-Todd, D. A., Renshaw, P. F., Smith, K. R., & Hanson, G. R. (2018). Increased risk of diseases of the basal ganglia and cerebellum in patients with a history of attention-deficit/hyperactivity disorder. *Neuropsychopharmacology*, *43*(13), 2548–2555.

Danielson, M. L., Bitsko, R. H., Ghandour, R. M., Holbrook, J. R., Kogan, M. D., & Blumberg, S. J. (2018). Prevalence of parent-reported ADHD diagnosis and associated treatment among U.S. children and adolescents, 2016. *Journal of Clinical Child and Adolescent Psychology*, *47*(2), 199–212.

del Campo, N., Fryer, T. D., Hong, Y. T., Smith, R., Brichard, L., Acosta-Cabronero, J., … Müller, U. (2013). A positron emission tomography study of nigro-striatal dopaminergic mechanisms underlying attention: Implications for ADHD and its treatment. *Brain*, *136*(11), 3252–3270.

Faraone, S. V., & Larsson, H. (2019). Genetics of attention deficit hyperactivity disorder. *Molecular Psychiatry*, *24*(4), 562–575.

Fischer, J., & Fischer, A. (1966). *The New Englanders of Orchard Town*. New York: John Wiley and Sons.

Gøtzsche, P. C. (2019). *Death of a Whistleblower and Cochrane's Moral Collapse*. People's Press.

Hoogman, M., Bralten, J., Hibar, D. P., Mennes, M., Zwiers, M. P., Schweren, L. S. J., … Franke, B. (2017). Subcortical brain volume differences in participants with attention deficit hyperactivity disorder in children and adults: A cross-sectional mega-analysis. *Lancet Psychiatry*, *4*(4), 310–319.

Jenkins, H. (Ed.). (1998). *The Children's Culture Reader*. New York: New York University Press.

Jensen, P. S., Arnold, L. E., Swanson, J. M., Vitiello, B., Abikoff, H. B., Greenhill, L. L., … Hur, K. (2007). 3-year follow-up of the 248 NIMH MTA study. *Journal of the American Academy of Child and Adolescent Psychiatry, 46*(8), 989–1002.

Joseph, J. (2006). *The Missing Gene: Psychiatry, Heredity, and the Fruitless Search for Genes.* New York: Algora Publishing.

Joseph, J. (2015). *The Trouble with Twin Studies: A Reassessment of Twin Research in the Social and Behavioral Sciences.* New York: Routledge.

Luk, S. L., & Leung, P. W. (1989). Conners' teacher's rating scale – a validity study in Hong Kong. *Journal of Child Psychology and Psychiatry, 30*(5), 785–793.

Mann, E. M., Ikeda, Y., Mueller, C. W., Takahashi, A., Tao, K. T., Humris, E., … Chin, D. (1992). Cross-cultural differences in rating hyperactive-disruptive behaviors in children. *American Journal of Psychiatry, 149*(11), 1539–1542.

Moncrieff, J., & Timimi, S. (2010). Is ADHD a valid diagnosis in adults? No. *British Medical Journal, 340,* 736–737.

Moncrieff, J., & Timimi, S. (2011). Critical analysis of the concept of adult attention deficit hyperactivity disorder. *The Psychiatrist, 35*(9), 334–338.

Odier, B. (2004). La psychiatrie à l'épreuve du scientisme. *L'information Psychiatrique, 80*(7), 557–565.

Rapoport, J. L., Buchsbaum, M. S., Zahn, T., Weingartner, H., Ludlow, C., & Mikkelsen, E. J. (1978). Dextroamphetamine: Cognitive and behavioral effects in normal prepubertal boys. *Science, 199*(4328), 560–563.

Rapoport, J. L., Buchsbaum, M. S., Zahn, T., Weingarten, H., Ludlow, C., & Mikkelsen, E. J. (1980). Dextroamphetamine: Its cognitive and behavioral effects in normal and hyperactive boys and normal men. *Archives of General Psychiatry, 37*(8), 933–943.

Singh, I. (2011). A disorder of anger and aggression: Children's perspectives on attention deficit/hyperactivity disorder in the UK. *Social Science & Medicine, 73*(6), 889–896.

Smith, M. (2012). *Hyperactive: The Controversial History of ADHD.* London: Reaktion Books.

Still, G. F. (1902). On some abnormal psychical conditions in children. *Lancet, 159*(4102), 1008–1012; (4103), 1077–1082; (4104), 1163–1168.

Storebø, O. J., Ramstad, E., Krogh, H. B., Nilausen, T. D., Skoog, M., Holmskov, M., … Gluud, C. (2015). Methylphenidate for children and adolescents with attention deficit hyperactivity disorder (ADHD). *Cochrane Database of Systematic Reviews, 2015*(11), CD009885.

Strauss, A., & Lehtinen, L. (1947). *Psychopathology and Education of the Brain Injured Child.* New York: Grune and Stratton.

The MTA Co-operative Group. (1999a). A 14-month randomized clinical trial of treatment strategies for attention deficit/hyperactivity disorder. *Archives of General Psychiatry, 56*(12), 1073–1086.

The MTA Co-operative Group. (1999b). Moderators and mediators of treatment response for children with attention-deficit/hyperactivity disorder. *Archives of General Psychiatry, 56*(12), 1088–1096.

Timimi, S. (2005). *Naughty Boys: Anti-Social Behaviour, ADHD and the Role of Culture.* London: Palgrave Macmillan.

Timimi, S. (2015). Attention deficit hyperactivity disorder is an example of bad medicine. *Australian and New Zealand Journal of Psychiatry, 49*(6), 575–576.

Timimi, S. (2017). Non-diagnostic based approaches to helping children who could be labelled ADHD and their families. *International Journal of Qualitative Studies on Health and Well-Being, 12*(sup1), 1298270.

Timimi, S. (2018a). Attention-deficit hyperactivity disorder: A critique of the concept. *Irish Journal of Psychological Medicine, 35*(3), 257–259.

Timimi, S. (2018b). Rebuttal to Dr Foreman's article on 'ADHD: Progress and controversy in diagnosis and treatment'. *Irish Journal of Psychological Medicine, 35*(3), 251–257.

Timimi, S., & 33 co-endorsers. (2004). A critique of the international consensus statement on ADHD. *Clinical Child and Family Psychology Review, 7*(1), 59–63.

Timimi, S., & Leo, J. (Eds.). (2009). *Rethinking ADHD: From Brain to Culture*. Basingstoke: Palgrave Macmillan.

Timimi, S., & Taylor, E. (2004). In Debate: ADHD is best understood as a cultural construct. *British Journal of Psychiatry, 184*(1), 8–9.

Timimi, S., & Timimi, L. (2015). The social construction of Attention Deficit Hyperactivity Disorder (ADHD). In M. O'Reilly (Ed.), *The Palgrave Handbook of Child Mental Health* (pp. 139–157). London: Palgrave Macmillan.

Whitaker, R., & Cosgrove, L. (2015). *Psychiatry under the Influence: Institutional Corruption, Social Injury, and Prescriptions for Reform*. New York: Palgrave Macmillan.

Whitely, M., Raven, M., Timimi, S., Jureidini, J., Phillimore, J., Leo, J., ... Landman, P. (2019). Annual Research Review: Attention deficit hyperactivity disorder late birthdate effect common in both high and low prescribing international jurisdictions: A systematic review. *The Journal of Child Psychology and Psychiatry, 60*(4), 380–391. doi: 10.111/jcpp.12991.

Williams, N. M., Zaharieva, I., Martin, A., Langley, K., Mantripragada, K., Fossdal, R., ... Thapar, A. (2010). Rare chromosomal deletions and duplications in attention-deficit hyperactivity disorder: A genome-wide analysis. *The Lancet, 376*(9750), 1401–1408.

Chapter 3

The problem with biomedical approaches and the necessity for psychoanalysis as exemplified by hyperactivity/ADHD

Sébastien Ponnou

***

This chapter proposes an enlightened critique of the problems of biomedical and standardized approaches to Attention Deficit Disorder with or without Hyperactivity (ADHD) in France. It argues for the necessity of psychoanalysis and its clinic in the treatment of ADHD children and their parents.

ADHD is considered the most common mental disorder in school-aged children (Sayal et al., 2018). For this reason, it has been the object of thousands of studies worldwide, the result being that our knowledge of ADHD has evolved considerably over time.

While initial investigations in the 1980s and 1990s suggested the existence of a biological etiology of ADHD, subsequent studies and meta-analyses have since refuted a causal impact. Thus, there are currently no neurological markers, genetic markers or biological tests to identify or confirm the diagnosis of hyperactivity (Dumas-Mallet & Gonon, 2020). Moreover, studies investigating the neurobiology or genetics of ADHD have proven to be so inconsistent and contradictory that the hypothesis of a biological etiology for hyperactivity diminishes as new research emerges.

As there are no biological markers or tests to confirm the diagnosis, the description of ADHD relies exclusively on evaluating behavioral symptoms, namely, an attention deficit with or without motor impulsivity and hyperactivity. For this reason, the prevalence of ADHD is intensely debated at the international level, with significant variations depending on countries, regions and the survey methods used (Ponnou, 2022; Polanczyk et al., 2014).

Similarly, recommendations for treatment vary considerably between countries (Sayal et al., 2018). In North America, drug treatment is recommended as the first line of treatment, whereas in most European countries, a psychotherapeutic, educational and social approach is officially preferred. In principle, medication is reserved for the most severe cases (Sayal et al., 2018).

In terms of medication, the only compound authorized in France for the treatment of ADHD is methylphenidate (MPH). It is marketed in a simple form (Ritalin®) and a delayed form (Ritalin-LP®, Concerta®, Quasym®, Medikinet®). MPH is

DOI: 10.4324/9781003584469-4

recommended for children aged 6 years and over "when psychological, educational, social and family corrective measures alone are insufficient" (ANSM, 2017). Prescription is subject to strict limitations and conditions of delivery. These include initial prescription and annual renewals carried out in a hospital setting by specialists (until September 2021), monthly renewals following specific prescription protocols and the identification of the pharmacist filling out the prescription (ANSM, 2017).

While biomedical research has produced limited results regarding the neurobiology, genetics and treatment of ADHD, numerous studies have shown the influence of the school system on the diagnosis and medication of children with ADHD. For example, in one city in the state of Virginia, 63% of schoolchildren who were one year ahead of their peers were treated with psychostimulants (LeFever, Dawson, & Morrow, 1999). In the general American population, the prevalence of ADHD varies relative to the month of birth, confirming that the youngest schoolchildren in their class are the most at risk (Elder, 2010; Evans, Morrill, & Parente, 2010). A Canadian study showed that the number of boys treated with a psychostimulant is 41% higher if they were born in December than if they were born in January. For girls, the rate is 77% (Morrow et al., 2012). Elsewhere, Elder (2010) shows that the hyperactive behavior of the youngest children in a class is more frequently judged pathological by their teachers than by their parents. American teachers are pressured by their superiors to report possible cases of ADHD to parents. Indeed, since a law was passed in 1990, American schools receive an additional allocation, which varies according to the county, for each child diagnosed, and the pharmaceutical industry provides teachers with the documentation necessary to identify potential cases (Phillips, 2006). Finally, schools are evaluated according to the performance of their students and are therefore encouraged to raise their academic level. A study comparing American states positively correlated the binding nature of these incentives with the prevalence of ADHD (Bokhari & Schneider, 2011). These surveys have been duplicated internationally, with the same phenomenon identified in Norway, Lombardy (Italy), Finland and the United Kingdom. Beyond the differences in the educational systems of these countries, the meta-analyses currently available support the hypothesis of an influence of the school system on the diagnosis of ADHD and on the medication of children (Holland & Sayal, 2019; Whitely et al., 2019).

Similarly, many environmental and social risk factors have been identified. These include exposure to toxic levels of lead (Needleman et al., 1979), premature birth (Linnet et al., 2006; Szatmari et al., 1990), severe child abuse, parents with mental disorders, poor interactions between parents and children (Biederman, Faraone, & Monuteaux, 2002; Biederman et al., 1995; Schneider & Eisenberg, 2006; Tallmadge & Barkley, 1983), low academic or economic level of the parents, and being part of a single-parent family or born of a teenage mother (Froehlich et al., 2007; Schneider & Eisenberg, 2006). Excessive exposure to television before the age of 3 years also seems to be particularly harmful to the development of a child's attention span (Christakis, 2009; Nikkelen et al., 2014; Beyens, Valkenburg, & Piotrowski, 2018).

Unfortunately, this type of study is lacking in France, meaning that questions concerning the prevalence of ADHD, drug prescription and the influence of academic and social factors on diagnosis and prescription are still highly controversial.

For this chapter dedicated to the problems of biomedical approaches to ADHD in France, we will focus on the following:

- The results of biomedical research in terms of the etiology and treatment of ADHD;
- The issues relating to the diagnosis and prevalence of ADHD in France;
- Medication with psychostimulants, in particular the inexorable increase in the consumption of MPH in children and adolescents;
- Academic and social factors related to the diagnosis of ADHD and to MPH medication in France;
- The scientific biases, media biases and conflicts of interest found in the information that is given to the general public and that can influence requests, practices and policies related to health.

It is essential that these elements be taken into account when addressing the principles and models that will underpin the care of children, adolescents and their families in France for the years to come.

1. Problems with biomedical approaches to ADHD

Contrary to popular belief, there is currently no neurological or genetic etiology for ADHD, as shown by François Gonon and Patrick Landman in previous chapters of this volume. In other words, there is no cause or biological test that can confirm the diagnosis of hyperactivity or justify the use of psychostimulants in children.

1.1. Is there scientific evidence for the neurological origin of ADHD?

Brain imaging studies published in the 1990s suggested that advances in neurobiology would soon allow diagnostic tools to be validated (Dougherty et al., 1999). Yet, there is currently no known test for ADHD (Weyandt, Swentosky, & Gudmundsdottir, 2013). Hundreds of structural and functional brain imaging studies have shown differences associated with ADHD, but none of these differences correspond to brain lesions. It is therefore impossible to label ADHD as a neurological disease or disorder. Furthermore, the differences are quantitatively small, contradictory, and only statistically significant when considering groups of children.

Some initial studies also suggested that the cause of ADHD was a dopamine deficit or the dysfunction of dopamine neurotransmitters. This perspective has been rigorously tested and refuted (Gonon, 2009). Thus, hypotheses regarding the neurological etiology of ADHD are now scientifically weak and dated (Gonon et al., 2012).

In addition to the inconsistency of the available results, the brain imaging studies cannot determine a potential cause of ADHD. In fact, it is impossible to determine whether the observations made relate to the cause or the consequence of a type of development specific to subjects with symptoms of hyperactivity.

1.2.   Is ADHD a genetic disease?

Initial studies also suggested a strong genetic etiology for ADHD. Subsequent studies and meta-analyses have largely refuted these associations or their causal impact. Currently, the best-established and most significant genetic risk factor is the association of ADHD with an allele of the gene coding for the dopamine D4 receptor (Gizer, Ficks, & Waldman, 2009). According to this meta-analysis, this risk factor is only 1.33 (Gizer et al., 2009). Specifically, this allele is present in 23% of children diagnosed with ADHD and only 17% of children in control groups (Shaw et al., 2007). This shows in essence an absence of effect and is thus inconclusive from a clinical point of view.

For example, a review of more than 300 genetic studies concluded that "the results from genetic studies regarding ADHD are still inconsistent and do not allow for any conclusions" (Li et al., 2014, p. 19). More generally, genetic studies – which are increasingly powerful and test millions of DNA variants in thousands of patients – all converge towards the same finding: the weight of genetic risk factors in the occurrence of mental disorders (including ADHD) decreases as the quality of the studies increases (Gaugler et al., 2014; Gonon, Dumas-Mallet, & Ponnou, 2019).

1.3.   Does psychostimulant treatment improve children's academic performance?

Studies in the 1990s predicted that treatment with psychostimulants would alleviate the symptoms of ADHD. The beneficial and apparently paradoxical effect of the treatment can in fact be explained otherwise: psychostimulants increase attention. The decrease of hyperactive and impulsive symptoms can thus be seen as the consequence of a longer attention span. However, according to several American studies that have followed very large cohorts of children over several years, psychostimulant treatment has no long-term benefits on the risks of academic failure, delinquency and substance abuse associated with ADHD (Currie, Stabile, & Jones, 2014; Gonon, Guilé, & Cohen, 2010; Humphreys, Eng, & Lee, 2013; Loe & Feldman, 2007; Sharpe, 2014; The MTA Cooperative Group, 1999).

1.4.   What are the contributions of biomedical research to the clinic?

These different elements call into question the extent to which biomedical research contributes to the ADHD clinic.

First, as there is no proven biological test or etiology for hyperactivity – as is the case with most "mental disorders" or "childhood disorders" – the diagnosis of ADHD is not based on scientific data but on heuristic conventions or uses whose reliability, relevance and clinical usefulness are debatable (Frances & Widiger, 2012).

Similarly, progress in biomedical research has not led to any major therapeutic breakthrough: no new class of psychotropic medication has been discovered for 50 years. Pharmaceutical companies are aware of this and have gradually closed their research units dedicated to psychiatry. Consequently, the drugs currently available are molecules or derivatives of molecules discovered between the 1950s and the 1970s thanks to clinical studies evaluated according to standard methods such as randomization or the use of placebos. This situation leads to at least two paradoxes, particularly in the case of ADHD:

- MPH, the most commonly prescribed drug treatment for ADHD internationally, including in France (Sayal et al., 2018), was synthesized in 1944 and patented in the 1950s, long before ADHD emerged as a diagnostic category. The approach to ADHD has been compromised by this extraordinary reversal of conventional clinical and medical logic (Canguilhem, 1966; Foucault, 1963): it is no longer a question of finding a treatment to cure the disease or of developing a therapy that relieves the patient's suffering, but of constructing the most suitable nosographic framework for the use of a given molecule.
- Similarly, the benefit/risk ratio of MPH is assessed independently of any causal logic. The prescription of psychostimulants cannot in any way be advocated on the basis of a biological etiology (for example, a deficit in dopamine neurotransmitters) since this hypothesis has been disproved. In other words, even if the treatment works and alleviates the symptoms of ADHD, the question of how and why the treatment works remains.

These observations concerning the problems of biomedical approaches to ADHD (and biological psychiatry in general; see Gonon, 2011) have been shared by leading figures in science who have been involved in biomedical research on mental disorders for decades.

For example, Steven Hyman, Director of the Stanley Center for Psychiatric Research, and Professor and Fellow of the Broad Institute at MIT and Harvard, considers that:

Although neuroscience has advanced in recent decades, the difficulties are such that the search for biological causes of mental disorders has largely failed.
(Hyman, 2018).

Similarly, Thomas Insel, in his book *Healing: Our Path from Mental Illness to Mental Health* says the following:

I have wrestled with mental illness as a parent, a scientist and a doctor physician for nearly half a century. Trained as a psychiatrist and working as a neuroscientist, I've spent the last four decades witnessing research breakthroughs on how the brain works in both health and disease. Ultimately, I became, for more than a decade, the "nation's psychiatrist", director of the National Institute of Mental Health (NIMH), overseeing more than $20 billion for mental health research. I helped President George W. Bush respond to school shootings and co-led President Barack Obama's Brain Initiative. I advised members of Congress on mental health care and worked with leaders in the Pentagon on suicide in the military. In short, it was my job to make a difference for Americans with mental illness. I should have been able to help us bend the curves for death and disability. But I didn't. Because I misunderstood the problem. Or maybe it's more accurate to say that the problem I was solving by supporting brilliant scientists and dedicated clinicians was not the problem that faced nearly fifteen million Americans living with serious mental illness.

(Insel, 2022a).

In a recent interview with the *New York Times* (2022b), Insel also stated that, for the most part, the advances in neuroscience had not yet benefited patients.

Finally, in a 2019 article entitled "Medicine and the mind—The consequences of psychiatry's identity crisis", published in the prestigious *New England Journal of Medicine*, Gardner and Kleinman stated that:

Ironically, although [the limitations of biological treatments] are widely recognized by experts in the field, the prevailing message to the public and the rest of medicine remains that the solution to psychological problems involves matching the "right" diagnosis with the "right" medication.

(Gardner & Kleinman, 2019, p. 1697).

The problem, according to Gardner and Kleinman in the *NEJM* (2019), is that even though there is no comprehensive biological understanding of either the causes or the treatments of psychiatric disorders, psychiatric diagnoses and medications proliferate under the banner of scientific medicine. The authors consider that this state of affairs influences training and reimbursement and does a great disservice to patients and practicing psychiatrists.

With these observations about the state of biomedical research on ADHD internationally, we now turn our attention to the situation in France in order to address how these pitfalls are characterized in terms of the prevalence, diagnosis and treatment of ADHD.

2.   The prevalence of hyperactivity/ADHD in France: archeology of a fake science

While no cases of ADHD were recorded in France before the 1990s, rates of occurrence very quickly reached pandemic levels: first one child per class, then one child in ten. The diagnosis of hyperactivity in that country began to emerge only after the introduction of psychostimulant medication (MPH) in 1995.

Between 2008 and 2011, the pharmaceutical industry (most notably Shire®, the laboratory which markets the most widely prescribed version of MPH in France) financed a telephone survey concluding that there was a high prevalence of ADHD in France (between 3.5% and 5.6% of all children). The results of this study are still widely disseminated by public authorities, health agencies, the media and professional journals. However, apart from an obvious conflict of interest, which is in itself quite problematic, the methodology upon which this research was based is questionable: it consisted of a telephone survey entrusted to non-specialist operators, trained on the fly, of a relatively small sample of the population (a little more than 1000 households). Now how is it possible to determine whether a child has hyperactivity/ADHD without having ever met or spoken to him or her? How can a reliable prevalence rate be inferred?

According to these highly questionable methodological criteria, the researchers estimated that 36 children (3.5%) aged between 6 and 12 years suffered from hyperactivity/ADHD, and that 22 children (2.2%) were treated with psychostimulants without being formally diagnosed (Lecendreux, Konofal, & Faraone, 2011, p. 517). The authors conclude that the prevalence rate of ADHD in France is between 3.5% and 5.6%. The study also shows that among the 3.5% of children diagnosed as hyperactive, 36.5% are also treated with MPH: the ratio of children diagnosed with ADHD who are treated with MPH in France is 36.5% (Lecendreux et al., 2011, p. 517). Consequently, the study points to an MPH prescription rate of 3.48% among children aged 6–12 years (2.2% + (3.5% × 0.365) = 3.48%).

However, a comparison of these data with the MPH consumption rates recorded in the French National Health Data System (*Système National des Données de Santé* or SNDS) for the entire French population showed that the results presented in the telephone study by Lecendreux and colleagues were 17 times higher than the actual prescriptions made by doctors. The analysis of health databases thus shows contradictions, inconsistencies and a clear overestimation of the results of the initial study supported by the drug industry. As a result, given what scientists know at this stage, the prevalence rate of ADHD in France has yet to be established (Ponnou, 2022; Ponnou & Haliday, 2021a, 2021b).

In general, the volatility of the prevalence rate of ADHD can be observed at the international level, with significant variations ranging from 0.4% to 16.6% of school-age children, and surveys pointing to exorbitant prevalence rates of 20% or even 25% of ADHD among children (Polanczyk et al., 2014). ADHD prevalence is estimated at 1% in Great Britain and 10% in the United States, but there again with significant variations from one state to another. Meta-analyses show that, as is the case in France, prevalence rates are determined by the research method used: clinical studies, telephone surveys or questionnaires given to parents and/or teachers. Unfortunately, these different types of surveys have many biases that call into question or even invalidate their scope: variations according to the diagnostic criteria, the scales and analysis grids used, sampling, the level of training of the investigators and the level of information of the respondents, taking into account the risks of comorbidity, diagnostic errors or social factors which can influence the diagnosis (Ponnou, 2022; Polanczyk et al., 2014). In short, far from being an exact science, studies on the prevalence of ADHD in France are a fake science.

3.   A steady increase in the use of psychostimulants in children

Let us now look at MPH consumption in children and adolescents in France. A recent survey of health databases covering 87% of the French population shows not only a steady increase in the use of psychostimulants in children, but also a systematic undermining of the regulatory conditions for prescribing them (Ponnou et al., 2022).

3.1.   Changes in MPH consumption among children and adolescents in France, and duration of treatment

A study carried out among all French children and adolescents (0–17 years) between 2010 and 2019 shows that MPH consumption more than doubled over those ten years: +56% for incidence,[1] and +116% for prevalence[2] (Ponnou et al., 2022). This general increase is part of a continuum, previous studies having already reported an increase of 65% between 2003 and 2005, and 135% between 2005 and 2011.

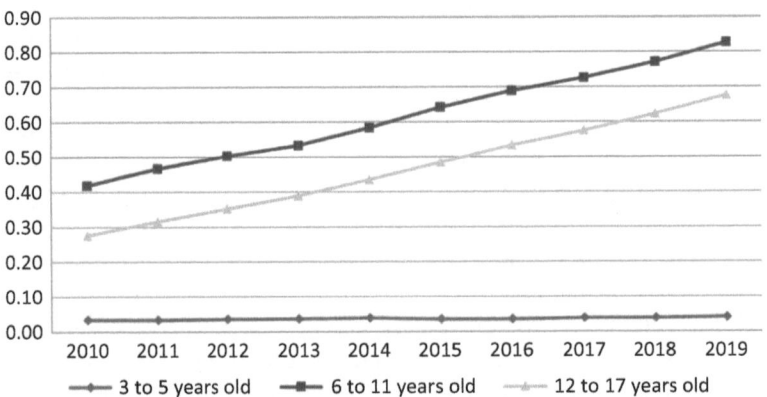

Changes in the prevalence rate of MPH prescription

This rate is expressed as a percentage of the general population for each age group and period.

This increase is coupled with a considerable lengthening of treatment durations: the median duration of consumption among 6-year-olds in 2011 was 5.5 years, and up to more than 8 years for 25% of them. Even more worrying is that the youngest children have the longest treatment times. These durations are not comparable to those highlighted in the 2000s: the median duration of MPH prescription in children in France in 2005 was 10.2 months (Knellwolf et al., 2008). Since the evolution of MPH consumption between 2010 and 2019 shows an increase in prevalence much higher than in incidence, it is likely that treatment durations will be significantly higher in 2019 than as per the data recorded in 2011.

Median durations of MPH treatment for patients with an initial prescription in 2011

Ages	Numbers of children	Median durations of treatment in days (years)
2	7	3077 (8.4)
3	44	1227 (3.4)
4	113	1991 (5.5)
5	338	1870 (5.1)
6	1069	1990 (5.5)
7	1352	1581 (4.3)
8	1406	1443 (4)
9	1359	1254 (3.4)
10	916	1089 (3)
11	875	757 (2.1)
12	845	680 (1.9)
13	669	552 (1.5)
14	488	412.5 (1.1)
15	346	279 (0.8)
16	255	387 (1.1)
17	168	248 (0.7)

3.2. Systematic undermining of regulatory conditions for prescribing

The analysis of health databases also shows a considerable number of prescriptions occurring outside the French marketing authorization (*Autorisation de mise sur le marché*, or AMM) and prescription recommendations.[3]

1) Contrary to the AMM recommendations, MPH is prescribed before the age of 6 years.
2) Treatment durations are particularly long and steadily increasing, while prescribing guidelines clearly recommend short-term use and regular re-evaluation of the drug's benefits.
3) Contrary to the regulatory obligations in force until 13 September 2021, 25% of initial prescriptions and 50% of annual renewals are not carried out by a hospital specialist.

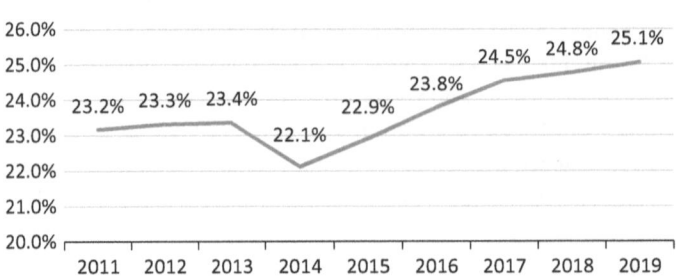

Evolution of out-of-hospital initial MPH prescriptions, 2011–2019

Renewal of prescription of incident patients in hospital in 2015, 2016 and 2017

Number of patients	Patients without hospital renewal at 1 year + 1 month	Patients without hospital renewal at 1 year + 2 months
31,942	16,921 (52.9%)	15,839 (49.6%)

4) Medical and psycho-educational follow-up of children does not always seem to be carried out satisfactorily: most children (84%) do not benefit from any medical consultation from the prescribing hospital service within 13 months following the initiation of treatment. Between 2010 and 2019, the number of consultations in a French medical-psychological-pedagogical center (*Centre Médico-Psycho-Pédagogique*, or CMPP)[4] decreased by 75%, while the prevalence of MPH use more than doubled. These results suggest that there is a risk of drug prescriptions replacing therapeutic and socio-educational practices.

CMPP visits among patients with an MPH prescription

Year	Patients	Visits	Visits/patient	Total patients	% total
2010	1305	21,083	16.16	31,453	4.1%
2011	1169	22,105	18.91	37,583	3.1%
2012	1244	23,963	19.26	42,282	2.9%
2013	1277	26,274	20.57	46,261	2.8%
2014	1292	27,171	21.03	51,041	2.5%
2015	1258	25,362	20.16	56,938	2.2%
2016	1301	26,073	20.04	62,028	2.1%
2017	1308	29,213	22.33	66,461	2.0%
2018	817	15,769	19.30	70,103	1.2%
2019	550	10,175	18.50	72,798	0.8%

5) Although MPH prescription in France is supposedly restricted to cases of ADHD, the molecule is in reality more widely prescribed. Furthermore, when a psychiatric diagnosis is actually made, it does not always correspond to the therapeutic indication defined by the AMM. The French summary of product characteristics (*Résumé des Caractéristiques du Produit*, or RCP) states that "psychostimulants are not intended for [...] patients with other primary psychiatric conditions [...]".[5]

6) A quarter (22.8%) of children and adolescents who take MPH also receive one or more other psychotropic drugs in the year following the initial prescription: neuroleptics (64.5%), anxiolytics (35.5%), antidepressants (16.2%), antiepileptics (11%), hypnotics (4.8%) and antiparkinsonians (3%).

    These co-prescriptions are often very far from AMM recommendations and are outside the recommendations of the French National Authority for Health (*Haute Autorité de Santé*, or HAS). The main molecules prescribed are derivatives or generic versions of risperidone (Risperdal® – 10.6%), hydroxyzine (Atarax® – 6%), cyamemazine (Tercian® – 3.9%) aripiprazole (Abilify® – 2.7%), sertraline (Zoloft® – 1.4%), valproic acid (Depakine® – 1.1%) and fluoxetine (Prozac® – 1%).

    Of those children who had been prescribed several psychotropic drugs in the year following the first MPH delivery, 63.5% had received two treatments (MPH and another psychotropic drug), 20.8% had received three psychotropic drugs, 8.5% had received four and 6.9% had been prescribed five or more psychotropic drugs. The co-prescription of other psychotropic drugs – especially antipsychotics – in combination with MPH poses serious health risks for the child and should be avoided (Libowitz & Nurmi, 2021).

4. The influence of the school system and social inequalities on the diagnosis of ADHD and the prescription of psychostimulants in children and adolescents in France

We will now consider the influence of the school system and social inequalities on ADHD diagnosis and the use of psychostimulants.

4.1. The influence of the school system on ADHD diagnosis and MPH prescription

The same research on ADHD diagnosis and MPH prescription in health databases shows that the diagnosis of hyperactivity is systematically correlated with the month of birth of the child, the youngest pupils in their class being the most likely to be diagnosed as hyperactive.

    Thus, in 2011, there were significantly more children diagnosed as hyperactive born in December (291) than in January (170). This can be observed over the period studied: in 2019, of the 4337 children identified as having ADHD as their main diagnosis in the health databases, 487 were born in December and 294 in January. Overall, children born in December are 55% more likely to be diagnosed with ADHD than their peers born in January (min. 41%, max. 71% over the period 2011–2019).

This influence of the school system reveals a social and demographic inequality that is all the more striking as it constitutes a pattern presiding over the diagnosis.

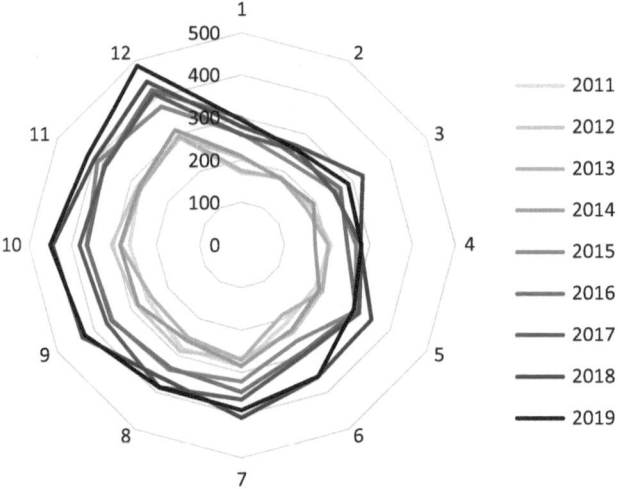

Month of birth of ADHD children who received an initial hospital diagnosis between 2011 and 2019

Similarly, French children and adolescents were 44%–60% more likely to be prescribed a psychostimulant treatment if they were born in December than if they were born in January (54% on average, over the whole period). Between 2010 and 2019, the number of initial treatments increased systematically over the months of the year in which children were born. This occurred gradually from January to December, only to fall sharply in January of the following year. Thus, a child's month of birth is significantly correlated not only with ADHD diagnosis but also with how the child is medicated.

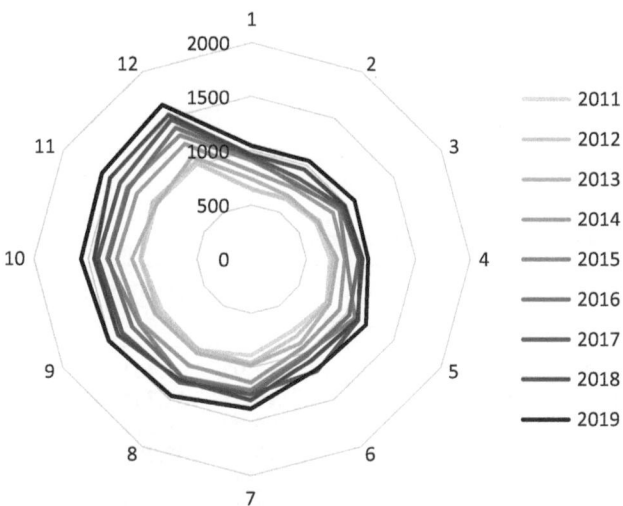

Children and adolescents treated with MPH by month of birth between 2011 and 2019

4.2. Socially determined diagnosis and prescription

Between 2010 and 2019, 35.2%–38.8% of children diagnosed with ADHD lived in families benefiting from the French universal health coverage (*Couverture Maladie Universelle*, or CMU) or complementary health insurance (CMU-C). However, according to the French National Institute of Statistics and Economic Studies (*Institut national de la statistique et des études économiques*, or INSEE), only 7.8% of the French population benefited from these health coverage plans. ADHD diagnosis was therefore much more frequent among children from the most disadvantaged families. If we also consider ADHD children who, in addition, come from a socially disadvantaged background, the percentage of children with social difficulties in the ADHD cohort was between 39.8% and 42.6% over the period.

Levels of social disadvantage among children and adolescents taking MPH

Year	CMU + CMU-C	%	CMU + social disadvantage diagnosis	%	Total population
2010	1217	38.3%	1305	41%	3181
2011	1388	38.5%	1501	41.7%	3602
2012	1591	38.8%	1734	42.3%	4100
2013	1400	37%	1527	40.4%	3780
2014	1520	38.5%	1667	42.2%	3950
2015	1765	35.6%	1971	39.8%	4956
2016	1944	36.2%	2211	41.2%	5373
2017	1845	35.2%	2096	40%	5243
2018	2200	36.9%	2538	42.6%	5957
2019	2211	35.4%	2580	41.4%	6238

Similarly, in 2019, 21.7% of children prescribed MPH lived in families benefiting from CMU or CMU-C. This rate was much higher than that for the allocation of these aids in the general population (7.8%). This trend increased between 2010 and 2019. If we also consider children treated with MPH and also coming from a socially disadvantaged background,[6] the percentage of children with social difficulties in the cohort who were prescribed MPH reaches 25.7%.

Levels of social disadvantage among children and adolescents taking MPH

Year	CMU + CMU-C %		CMU + social disadvantage diagnosis	%	Total population
2010	4240	14.4%	5254	**17.9%**	29,402
2011	4869	14.9%	6008	**18.3%**	32,762
2012	5475	15.2%	6733	**18.7%**	36,014
2013	5918	15.1%	7326	**18.7%**	39,212
2014	6833	15.7%	8380	**19.3%**	43,477
2015	7762	16.1%	9455	**19.6%**	48,206
2016	8705	16.6%	11,088	**21.1%**	52,574
2017	10,512	18.5%	12,983	**22.9%**	56,778
2018	12,495	20.6%	15,017	**24.7%**	60,762
2019	14,181	21.7%	16,782	**25.7%**	65,395

5.   Accounting for the evolution of psychostimulant prescription in children: analysis of scientific biases, media biases and conflicts of interest concerning hyperactivity/ADHD in France

How can the evolution in the prescription and care practices for children and adolescents in France be accounted for? Several studies have shown that most discourse surrounding hyperactivity does not reflect international consensus: there exist scientific biases, media biases and conflicts of interest, all of which produce systematic distortions of the image of ADHD in the media and among the general public in France.

5.1.   Scientific and media biases having an impact on the general public's image of ADHD

There are documented scientific and media biases that may account for the systematic distortions between international consensus and the information disseminated among the general public concerning ADHD in France. We will now take two examples from neurobiology and children's academic performance, provided by François Gonon in two recent articles (Dumas-Mallet & Gonon, 2020; Gonon, Dumas-Mallet, & Ponnou, 2019).

One of the most blatant cases of scientific fraud concerning hyperactivity is perhaps the study by Dougherty and colleagues, published in 1999 in the prestigious journal *The Lancet*. The study concluded that the brain level of the dopamine transporter is 70% higher in hyperactive patients. The dopamine transporter is a membrane protein that regulates neurotransmission involving dopamine. This article was widely covered by the scientific literature and the mainstream press because it claimed to explain the cause of ADHD and the rationale for the treatment of it, since psychostimulants inhibit this transporter. What the authors failed to mention in the 1999 article is that 4 of their 6 patients had previously received long-term treatment with a psychostimulant, information that was not published until 2005. Subsequent studies have shown that dopamine transporter levels are similar in control subjects and untreated patients with ADHD and that prolonged treatment with psychostimulants increases this rate. This is a clear case of fraud, and one which has contributed to conveying the idea of neurological causality and supporting the use of psychostimulants in children with ADHD. However, the study by Dougherty and colleagues (1999) was covered by 22 press articles in the week following its publication. Between 2000 and 2010, 11 subsequent studies were conducted. All of these studies have largely downgraded, if not refuted, the findings of the original study, rejecting the hypothesis of neurological causation of ADHD and, consequently, the benefits of psychostimulant treatment. The 2012 meta-analysis also concluded that there was no difference in dopamine transporter levels between diagnosed ADHD patients and controls, thus refuting the hypothesis and observations of the original study (Fusar-Poli et al., 2012). However, of the 11 subsequent studies, only 1 was covered in the press (by a mere 3 articles, for that matter) and none of the articles stated that the initial study, although covered by their publication, had been contradicted by this subsequent study.

Another example is the study by Barbaresi and colleagues (2007), which reports that treating children with ADHD with a psychostimulant neither improves their reading performance nor reduces their risk of early school leaving. However, on the sole basis of a class repetition rate that is slightly lower, they conclude that this treatment improves their school performance in the long term. This serious form of distortion, referred to as spin, consists of a glaring inconsistency between the observations described in the article and the conclusion drawn at the end of the article and/or in the summary. Unfortunately, this practice is widespread in the field of biomedical research. In this case, it gives rise to the hope that the use of psychostimulants will improve academic performance, an assertion that has no scientific basis. Yet the conclusion of the study by Barbaresi and colleagues was simply reproduced in 20 of the 21 articles in the English-language press that covered the study. Only the *Guardian* article correctly described all the observations and therefore criticized the conclusion drawn in the study. This type of hypothesis, which denies both the child's desire to know and his or her involvement in complex learning processes, is nothing less than absurd. Unfortunately, these scientific distortions are all the more worrying as they are amplified by media bias, which only increases their effects (Dumas-Mallet & Gonon, 2020; Gonon, Dumas-Mallet, & Ponnou, 2019).

5.2. Distortions in the scientific discourse surrounding ADHD in the media

These examples are not isolated cases, nor are they restricted to the English-language literature. Indeed, recent studies published in international journals have compared the state of scientific knowledge with the discourse surrounding ADHD in the French media. These studies have focused on the three issues presented in the first part of this chapter:

- Can ADHD be described as a neurological or neurodevelopmental disorder?
- Is ADHD a genetic disorder?
- Does MPH treatment improve students' academic performance?

However, the results obtained showed that more than 87% of the information presented on television, 83% of the information disseminated by the press and 94% of the data presented on the internet concerning hyperactivity/ADHD contradict international scientific consensus (Bourdaa et al., 2015; Ponnou & Gonon, 2017; Ponnou, Haliday, & Gonon, 2020).

Level of distortion of scientific consensus on ADHD (neurology, genetics, medication and academic failure) in French TV programs, press articles and websites

	Media		
	Television	Press	Internet
General data			
Number of publications	60	159	50
First consensus: Neurologic or neurodevelopmental etiology for ADHD/Imaging diagnosis			
Against the consensus	6	26	27
In favor of the consensus	1	5	1
Both opinions	2	12	4
Second consensus: genetic etiology for ADHD			
Against the consensus	11	8	8
In favor of the consensus	2	5	1
Both opinions	3	12	11
Third consensus: Drug effects on school achievement			
Against the consensus	16	11	3
In favor of the consensus	3	4	1
Both opinions	3	2	4
Cumulative data			
Total opinions expressed	47	85	57
Against the consensus	33 (70.21%)	45 (52.94%)	38 (66.67%)
In favor of the consensus	6 (12.77%)	14 (16.47%)	3 (5.26%)
Both opinions	8 (17.02%)	26 (30.59%)	19 (33.33%)
Cumulative data against the consensus	**41/47 (87.23%)**	**71/85 (83.53%)**	**54/57 (94.74%)**

For example, on the website of one French association dedicated to ADHD, the following can be found:

Attention Deficit Hyperactivity Disorder (ADHD) is a biological brain condition likely caused by an imbalance in certain neurotransmitters in the brain, that is, the substances used to send signals between nerve cells.

(www.tdah-france.fr)

Another example can be found in the famous program "Allô Docteur" on the channel France 5, which, on 11 March 2010, broadcast a program on hyperactivity in children:[7]

ADHD is a neurological disease that affects the transmission of information in certain areas of the brain.

("Allô Docteur", broadcast on 11 March 2010)

Using brain imaging published in an article comparing adult dopamine transporter levels from a specific binding by cocaine diffusion (Volkow et al., 2007, p. 1184), the presenters explain the following:

You can see [at the top] the two little orange crescents. This is the area that releases dopamine. This is a normal case. And then you see [at the bottom] a case of ADHD. There is a little less dopamine secreted. As a result, the transmission of the nerve impulse cannot take place normally.

("Allô Docteur", broadcast on 11 March 2010)

François Gonon, a neurobiologist and director of research at the *Centre National de la Recherche Scientifique* (CNRS), has shown that this was a serious misuse of scientific discourse: contrary to the information broadcast in the program, these are not images of children's brains, but of adults' brains. Moreover, the methodological aspects of the study (the measurement of the level of dopamine transporters from a specific binding by cocaine diffusion (C11)) are not explained, whereas this information is crucial since the measurement of dopamine transporter levels is in this case conditioned by cocaine diffusion. Inferring from this that there is a dysfunction of the dopamine neurotransmitters in ADHD children – which incidentally has been refuted in the scientific literature (Gonon, 2009; Gonon et al., 2012) – is absurd.

Unfortunately, approximations or exaggerations of this type abound in the French media, contributing to the dissemination of partial, biased or erroneous information in favor of biomedical and medicinal approaches to hyperactivity.

5.3. Conflicts of interest and the influence of the pharmaceutical industry

In addition to scientific and media bias, the international literature regularly mentions the influence of pharmaceutical companies on care policies and practices for hyperactive children (Schwarz, 2017).

In France, the drug industry has largely contributed to the spread of these scientific biases and distortions. First, it financed the study concluding that there was a high prevalence of ADHD (between 3.5% and 5.6% in 2008), even though the data provided to support this conclusion were highly questionable.

The pharmaceutical industry has also financed the association Hyper-Super ADHD France, which advocates a biomedical approach to ADHD. However, interventions by experts or members of ADHD France, or references to the association's website, are particularly well represented in the media. This contributes to the distortions we have mentioned and suggests that a handful of experts exert significant influence on the general public. In general, these distortions shape discourse and have an impact on requests for care, professional practices and even health policies.

Furthermore, the association ADHD France – despite being subject to several types of conflicts of interest with the drug industry (subsidies, prices, even members of the scientific committee who are themselves subject to conflicts of interest) – directly influences health policies. For instance, the association contributes to the drafting of the HAS recommendations of good practice. On the grounds that access to treatment is difficult, ADHD France has also submitted several referrals to the health authorities in order to rescind the obligation requiring that an initial prescription of MPH be issued by a hospital practitioner.[8]

However, contrary to the arguments put forward by ADHD France, this obligation has never constituted an obstacle to the prescription of MPH. On the contrary, it has been designed to ensure the follow-up and support of children and their parents. The abolition of this obligation in September 2021, when weighed against the inexorable increase in consumption and non-compliance with prescription recommendations, bears witness to the real influence of the drug industry on mental health practices and policies in France. It all but guarantees the continued increase in the consumption of psychostimulants in children and adolescents.

These conflicting interests do not concern hyperactivity alone: the president of the Hyper-Super association also sits on the French National Council for Autism Spectrum Disorders and Neurodevelopmental Disorders (*Conseil national des Troubles du Spectre Autistique et des Troubles du Neuro-développement*), which ensures the shared monitoring of the national strategy for autism 2018–2022.

Finally, another type of conflict of interest concerns the sponsoring of hospital services by the pharmaceutical industry. (See for example https://u2peanantes.files .wordpress.com/2018/05/v5-maquette-tdah-3-nantes.pdf.)

Clearly, there are networks and mechanisms of influence which undermine ADHD research in France and internationally. These persist in the face of all scientific arguments, to the detriment of the interests of children and their families, and through the very associations that are supposed to represent them.

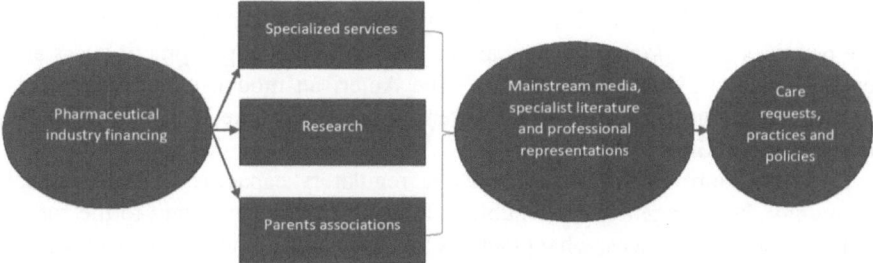

Conflicts of interest and the influence of the pharmaceutical industry on care requests and practices

6. Conclusion

In terms of etiology, diagnosis and therapy, advances in biomedical research on ADHD remain limited. Numerous studies highlight the following issues: an inexorable increase in the consumption of psychostimulants by children and adolescents in France; an increase in the duration of treatment and an almost systematic undermining of the regulatory conditions for prescription (prescriptions before the age of six, particularly long treatments, prescriptions outside an ADHD diagnosis and for other psychiatric diagnoses, co-prescriptions of other psychotropic drugs in combination with MPH, and non-compliance with the regulations surrounding initial prescription and subsequent renewals); the undermining of the conditions in which ADHD children are monitored and supported; and the proven risk of systematically substituting first-line psychotherapeutic, educational and social practices by medicinal treatment.

These issues are further compounded by the influence of the school system and of social disadvantage on ADHD diagnosis and MPH prescription, which point to a proven risk of medication of children according to age or social background. In addition to these examples of discrimination, there exist breaches of those prescription regulations that forge the democratic pact between citizens and their health system. Faced with this situation, neither the AMM, nor the recommendations or reminder letters from the ANSM, nor the warnings from researchers or health professionals who have been denouncing these abuses for many years seem to have been heard (Bursztejn et al., 2004).

This situation is associated with multiple scientific biases, media biases and conflicts of interest that can influence not only the image the public has of ADHD, but also the requests, the practices and even the policies related to the care of ADHD children in France.

Can we expect any benefits from the increasing medication of children's behavioral problems and from the progressive deregulation of the prescription of psychostimulants and even psychotropic drugs for young patients? Can children, adolescents and their families find better support from such medication? Can care practices be improved by it? Can the link between people, practitioners and health services be strengthened by it? The American model, which epitomizes the medicalization of psychological suffering, shows that the answer to all these questions is no (Gonon, 2011).

These questions raise doubts about the regulatory capacities of the medical community, health agencies and public authorities. They also bring to the fore a number of societal choices: what practices and what care model do we want for our children and the next generations? At the very least, these sensitive and complex issues deserve an informed and open scientific, political and public debate. This is all the more important in France, where psychological care, educational practices and social intervention are culturally ingrained in people's mentalities. These have proved their worth in clinical practice and constitute a specificity of French psychiatry and psychopathology. Now is the time to focus on the implementation of these practices. That is why we strongly advocate psychoanalysis and, with it, the preeminence of the subject, of speaking and of creativity.

Notes

1 Incidence refers to the number of new cases of a health phenomenon over a given period, in this case the number of new prescriptions of MPH per year between 2010 and 2019.
2 Prevalence refers to the total number of cases for a health phenomenon over a given period, in this case the total consumption of MPH per year among 0- to 17-year-olds between 2010 and 2019.
3 In France, the AMM is granted by the French Agency for the Safety of Health Products (*Agence nationale de sécurité du médicament et des produits de santé*, or ANSM) after a specific procedure to assess the benefit/risk ratio of a drug. This authorization is sometimes accompanied by conditions and prescription recommendations, as is the case for MPH.
4 The French medical-psychological-pedagogical centers (*Centres Médico-Psycho-Pédagogique*, or CMPPs) are reference structures providing psychosocial support for the child and the family.
5 From https://agence-prd.ansm.sante.fr/php/ecodex/rcp/R0141880.htm. Accessed 13 June 2021.
6 The diagnoses of disadvantage are listed in the International Classification of Diseases under the heading "Persons with potential health hazards related to socioeconomic and psychosocial circumstances". We referred to the following diagnoses: problems related to education and literacy; problems related to employment and unemployment; occupational exposure to risk factors; problems related to physical environment; problems related to housing and economic circumstances; problems related to social environment; problems related to negative life events in childhood; other problems related to upbringing; other problems related to primary support group, including

family circumstances; problems related to certain psychosocial circumstances; problems related to other psychosocial circumstances.

7 https://www.allodocteurs.fr/actualite-sante-l-hyperactivite-une-veritable-maladie _1961.html

8 https://www.tdah-france.fr/Fin-de-la-Prescription-Initiale-hospitaliere-PIH-pour-le -methylphenidate.html

References

Agence Nationale de Sécurité du Médicament (ANSM). (2017). Méthylphénidate: données d'utilisation et de sécurité d'emploi en France. https://archive.ansm.sante.fr/var/ansm _site/storage/original/application/b2137a9c7ec0a6113a7b8cf9c504384c.pdf

Barbaresi, W. J., Katusic, S. K., Colligan, R. C., Weaver, A. L., & Jacobsen, S. J. (2007). Long-term school outcomes for children with attention-deficit/hyperactivity disorder: A population-based perspective. *Journal of Developmental & Behavioral Pediatrics, 28*(4), 265–273.

Beyens, I., Valkenburg, P. M., & Piotrowski, J. T. (2018). Screen media use and ADHD-related behaviors: Four decades of research. *Proceedings of the National Academy of Sciences USA, 115*(40), 9875–9881.

Biederman, J., Faraone, S. V., & Monuteaux, M. C. (2002). Differential effect of environmental adversity by gender: Rutter's index of adversity in a group of boys and girls with and without ADHD. *The American Journal of Psychiatry, 159*(9), 1556–1562.

Biederman, J., Milberger, S., Faraone, S. V., Kiely, K., Guite, J., Mick, E., … Reed, E. (1995). Family-environment risk factors for attention-deficit hyperactivity disorder. A test of Rutter's indicators of adversity. *Archives of General Psychiatry, 52*(6), 464–470.

Bokhari, F. A., & Schneider, H. (2011). School accountability laws and the consumption of psychostimulants. *Journal of Health Economics, 30*(2), 355–372. doi: 10.1016/j. jhealeco.2011.01.007

Bourdaa, M., Konsman, J. P., Secail, C., Venturini, T., Veyrat-Masson, I., & Gonon, F. (2015). Does television reflect the evolution of scientific knowledge? The case of attention deficit hyperactivity disorder coverage on French TV. *Public Understanding of Science, 24*(2), 200–209.

Bursztejn, C., Chanseau, J. C., Geissmann, C., Golse, B., & Houzel, D. (2004). Ne bourrez pas les enfants de psychotropes! *Enfances & Psy*, (1), 42–45.

Canguilhem, G. (1966). *Le normal et le pathologique*. Paris: Presses Universitaires de France.

Christakis, D. A. (2009). The effects of infant media usage: What do we know and what should we learn? *Acta Paediatrica, 98*(1), 8–16.

Currie, J., Stabile, M., & Jones, L. (2014). Do stimulant medications improve educational and behavioral outcomes for children with ADHD? *Journal of Health Economics, 37*, 58–69.

Dougherty, D. D., Bonab, A. A., Spencer, T. J., Rauch, S. L., Madras, B. K., & Fischman, A. J. (1999). Dopamine transporter density in patients with attention deficit hyperactivity disorder. *Lancet, 354*(9196), 2132–2133.

Dumas-Mallet, E., & Gonon, F. (2020). Messaging in biological psychiatry: Misrepresentations, their causes, and potential consequences. *Harvard Review of Psychiatry, 28*(6), 395–403.

Elder, T. E. (2010). The importance of relative standards in ADHD diagnoses: Evidence based on exact birth dates. *Journal of Health Economics, 29*(5), 641–656. doi: 10.1016/j.jhealeco.2010.06.003

Evans, W. N., Morrill, M. S., & Parente, S. T. (2010). Measuring inappropriate medical diagnosis and treatment in survey data: The case of ADHD among school-age children. *Journal of Health Economics, 29*(5), 657–673. doi: 10.1016/j.jhealeco.2010.07.005

Foucault, M. (1963). *Naissance de la Clinique*. Paris: Presses Universitaires de France.

Frances, A. J., & Widiger, T. (2012). Psychiatric diagnosis: Lessons from the DSM-IV past and cautions for the DSM-5 future. *Annual Review of Clinical Psychology, 8*, 109–130.

Froehlich, T. E., Lanphear, B. P., Epstein, J. N., Barbaresi, W. J., Katusic, S. K., & Kahn, R. S. (2007). Prevalence, recognition, and treatment of attention-deficit/hyperactivity disorder in a national sample of US children. *Archives of Pediatrics & Adolescent Medicine, 161*(9), 857–864.

Fusar-Poli, P., Rubia, K., Rossi, G., Sartori, G., & Balottin, U. (2012). Striatal dopamine transporter alterations in ADHD: Pathophysiology or adaptation to psychostimulants? A meta-analysis. *The American Journal of Psychiatry, 169*(3), 264–272.

Gardner, C., & Kleinman, A. (2019). Medicine and the mind—the consequences of psychiatry's identity crisis. *The New England Journal of Medicine, 381*(18), 1697–1699.

Gaugler, T., Klei, L., Sanders, S. J., Bodea, C. A., Goldberg, A. P., Lee, A. B., ... Buxbaum, J. D. (2014). Most genetic risk for autism resides with common variation. *Nature Genetics, 46*(8), 881–885.

Gizer, I. R., Ficks, C., & Waldman, I. D. (2009). Candidate gene studies of ADHD: A meta-analytic review. *Human Genetics, 126*(1), 51–90.

Gonon, F. (2009). The dopaminergic hypothesis of attention-deficit/hyperactivity disorder needs re-examining. *Trends in Neuroscience, 32*(1), 2–8.

Gonon, F. (2011). La psychiatrie biologique: une bulle spéculative? *Esprit*, (Novembre), 54–73.

Gonon, F., Dumas-Mallet, E., & Ponnou, S. (2019). La couverture médiatique des observations scientifiques concernant les troubles mentaux. *Les Cahiers du journalisme, 2*(3), R45–R63.

Gonon, F., Guilé, J. M., & Cohen, D. (2010). Le trouble déficitaire de l'attention avec hyperactivité: données récentes des neurosciences et de l'expérience nord-américaine. *Neuropsychiatrie de l'enfance et de l'adolescence, 58*(5), 273–281.

Gonon, F., Konsman, J. P., Cohen, D., & Boraud, T. (2012). Why most biomedical findings echoed by newspapers turn out to be false: The case of Attention Deficit Hyperactivity Disorder. *PLoS ONE, 7*(9), e44275.

Holland, J., & Sayal, K. (2019). Relative age and ADHD symptoms, diagnosis and medication: A systematic review. *European Child & Adolescent Psychiatry, 28*(11), 1417–1429. https://doi.org/10.1007/s00787-018-1229-6

Humphreys, K. L., Eng, T., & Lee, S. S. (2013). Stimulant medication and substance use outcomes: A meta-analysis. *JAMA Psychiatry, 70*(7), 740–749.

Hyman, S. E. (2018). The daunting polygenicity of mental illness: Making a new map. *Philosophical Transactions of the Royal Society B: Biological Sciences, 373*(1742), 20170031.

Insel, T. (2022a). *Healing: Our Path from Mental Illness to Mental Health*. New York: Penguin Press.

Insel, T. (2022b). The 'Nation's Psychiatrist' takes stock, with frustration. *The New York Times*, February 22.

Knellwolf, A. L., Deligne, J., Chiarotti, F., Auleley, G. R., Palmieri, S., Boisgard, C. B., … & Autret-Leca, E. (2008). Prevalence and patterns of methylphenidate use in French children and adolescents. *European Journal of Clinical Pharmacology, 64*(3), 311–317.

Lecendreux, M., Konofal, E., & Faraone, S. V. (2011). Prevalence of attention deficit hyperactivity disorder and associated features among children in France. *Journal of Attention Disorders, 15*(6), 516–524.

LeFever, G. B., Dawson, K. V., & Morrow, A. L. (1999). The extent of drug therapy for attention deficit-hyperactivity disorder among children in public schools. *American Journal of Public Health, 89*(9), 1359–1364.

Li, Z., Chang, S. H., Zhang, L. Y., Gao, L., & Wang, J. (2014). Molecular genetic studies of ADHD and its candidate genes: A review. *Psychiatry Research, 219*(1), 10–24. doi:10.1016/j.psychres.2014.05.005

Libowitz, M. R., & Nurmi, E. L. (2021). The burden of antipsychotic-induced weight gain and metabolic syndrome in children. *Frontiers in Psychiatry, 12*, 623681.

Linnet, K. M., Wisborg, K., Agerbo, E., Secher, N. J., Thomsen, P. H., & Henriksen, T. B. (2006). Gestational age, birth weight, and the risk of hyperkinetic disorder. *Archives of Disease in Childhood, 91*(8), 655–660.

Loe, I. M., & Feldman, H. M. (2007). Academic and educational outcomes of children with ADHD. *Journal of Pediatric Psychology, 32*(6), 643–654.

Morrow, R. L., Garland, E. J., Wright, J. M., Maclure, M., Taylor, S., & Dormuth, C. R. (2012). Influence of relative age on diagnosis and treatment of attention-deficit/hyperactivity disorder in children. *Canadian Medical Association Journal, 184*(7), 755–762. doi: 10.1503/cmaj.111619

Needleman, H. L., Gunnoe, C., Leviton, A., Reed, R., Peresie, H., Maher, C., & Barrett, P. (1979). Deficits in psychologic and classroom performance of children with elevated dentine lead levels. *The New England Journal of Medicine, 300*(13), 689–695. doi: 10.1056/nejm197903293001301

Nikkelen, S. W., Valkenburg, P. M., Huizinga, M., & Bushman, B. J. (2014). Media use and ADHD-related behaviors in children and adolescents: A meta-analysis. *Developmental Psychology, 50*(9), 2228–2241.

Phillips, C. B. (2006). Medicine goes to school: Teachers as sickness brokers for ADHD. *PLoS Medicine, 3*(4), e182. doi: 10.1371/journal.pmed.0030182

Polanczyk, G. V., Willcutt, E. G., Salum, G. A., Kieling, C., & Rohde, L. A. (2014). ADHD prevalence estimates across three decades: An updated systematic review and meta-regression analysis. *International Journal of Epidemiology, 43*(2), 434–442.

Ponnou, S. (2022). Prévalence, diagnostic et médication de l'hyperactivité/TDAH en France. *Annales Médico Psychologiques, 180*(10), 995–999.

Ponnou, S., & Gonon, F. (2017). How French media have portrayed ADHD to the lay public and to social workers. *International Journal of Qualitative Studies on Health and Well-Being, 12*(sup1), 1298244.

Ponnou, S., & Haliday, H. (2021a). ADHD diagnosis and drug use estimates in France: A case for using health care insurance data. *Journal of Attention Disorders, 25*(10), 1347–1350. https://doi.org/10.1177/1087054720905664

Ponnou, S., & Haliday, H. (2021b). ADHD diagnosis and drug use estimates in France: A case for using health care insurance data – a response to Drs. Ramus and Peyre. *Journal of Attention Disorders*, *25*(11), 1634–1636.

Ponnou, S., Haliday, H., & Gonon, F. (2020). Where to find accurate information on attention-deficit hyperactivity disorder? A study of scientific distortions among French websites, newspapers, and television programs. *Health*, *24*(6), 684–700.

Ponnou, S., Haliday, H., Thomé, B., & Gonon, F. (2022). La prescription de méthylphénidate chez l'enfant et l'adolescent en France: caractéristiques et évolution entre 2010 et 2019. *Neuropsychiatrie de l'Enfance et de l'Adolescence*, *70*(3), 122–131.

Sayal, K., Prasad, V., Daley, D., Ford, T., & Coghill, D. (2018). ADHD in children and young people: Prevalence, care pathways, and service provision. *The Lancet Psychiatry*, *5*(2), 175–186.

Schneider, H., & Eisenberg, D. (2006). Who receives a diagnosis of attention-deficit/hyperactivity disorder in the United States elementary school population? *Pediatrics*, *117*(4), 601–609.

Schwarz, A. (2017). *ADHD Nation: Children, Doctors, Big Pharma, and the Making of an American Epidemic*. New York: Simon and Schuster.

Sharpe, K. (2014). Medication: The smart-pill oversell. *Nature*, *506*(7487), 146–149.

Shaw, P., Gornick, M., Lerch, J., Addington, A., Seal, J., Greenstein, D., ... Rapoport, J. L. (2007). Polymorphisms of the dopamine D4 receptor, clinical outcome, and cortical structure in attention-deficit/hyperactivity disorder. *Archives of General Psychiatry*, *64*(8), 921–931.

Szatmari, P., Saigal, S., Rosenbaum, P., Campbell, D., & King, S. (1990). Psychiatric disorders at five years among children with birthweights less than 1000g: A regional perspective. *Developmental Medicine & Child Neurology*, *32*(11), 954–962.

Tallmadge, J., & Barkley, R. A. (1983). The interactions of hyperactive and normal boys with their fathers and mothers. *Journal of Abnormal Child Psychology*, *11*(4), 565–579.

The MTA Cooperative Group. (1999). A 14-month randomized clinical trial of treatment strategies for attention-deficit/hyperactivity disorder. *Archives of General Psychiatry*, *56*(12), 1073–1086.

Volkow, N. D., Wang, G. J., Newcorn, J., Fowler, J. S., Telang, F., Solanto, M. V., ... & Pradhan, K. (2007). Brain dopamine transporter levels in treatment and drug naïve adults with ADHD. *Neuroimage*, *34*(3), 1182–1190.

Weyandt, L., Swentosky, A., & Gudmundsdottir, B. G. (2013). Neuroimaging and ADHD: fMRI, PET, DTI findings, and methodological limitations. *Developmental Neuropsychology*, *38*(4), 211–225.

Whitely, M., Raven, M., Timimi, S., Jureidini, J., Phillimore, J., Leo, J., ... & Landman, P. (2019). Annual Research Review: Attention deficit hyperactivity disorder late birthdate effect common in both high and low prescribing international jurisdictions: A systematic review. *The Journal of Child Psychology and Psychiatry*, *60*(4), 380–391.

Chapter 4

The hyperactive child, an unusual collective myth

Pascal-Henri Keller

***

1. The turbulent child: two cultures, two orientations

The years 1925 and 1937 mark the history of scientific interest in certain child behaviors that adults consider problematic, mainly that of agitation. From the adult's point of view, any phenomenon that opposes his or her power to mobilize the child's attention, especially when it comes to learning, is problematic. When an adult fails to sustain a child's attention, that child is said to be "turbulent". In 1925 the psychologist Henri Wallon wrote his doctoral thesis on the subject, and in 1937 Charles Bradley, an American pediatrician, discovered by chance the positive effects of benzedrine on this disorder. And it was Bradley who, so to speak, developed the first official psychostimulant for children in the United States who were not suited to school (Strohl, 2011). Around the same time in France, Henri Wallon opened up a whole field of research in child psychology based on his thesis (Wallon, 1984).

In short, Wallon described the psychic development of the child as a succession of stages separated by crises during which he progressively develops the intellectual tools to approach his external environment effectively. According to Wallon, the opposition of the child to this environment represents the usual mode of passage from one stage to another. Without this opposition, the child finds it difficult to feel truly independent of the environment on which he has depended entirely and on which he asserts himself through opposition. Being aware of the phases of the child's development, including those during which he opposes everyone around him, is supposed to enlighten parents, caregivers and teachers. In the end, the publication of Wallon's work made it clear that the instability of the child is less an organic disease than a psychological developmental characteristic.

A different strategy was adopted by certain American pediatricians in the hope of bringing into line children who manifested their opposition, be it with their family or at school. Their behavior was interpreted as the sign of a disease: the treatment that would make it disappear therefore had to be applied. Starting from these

DOI: 10.4324/9781003584469-5

assumptions, and with no other ambition than to advocate behavioral efficiency, this current of American pediatrics adopted an attitude that consisted in continually striving towards a single goal: that of eliminating this awkward symptom.

2. Children with behavioral tendencies, the DSM and Ritalin®

Nearly a century later, where do things stand? Has the new tool of world psychiatry proved Bradley right against Wallon? By officially describing Attention Deficit Disorder with or without Hyperactivity (ADHD), the Diagnostic and Statistical Manual of Mental Disorders (DSM) now establishes that what is responsible for the restless and oppositional behavior of children worldwide is indeed a genuine disease. It is all the easier to believe in this "disease" as its "discovery" is accompanied by the development of drug treatments that are said to cure it, including the famous Ritalin®.

But if the diagnosis of this pathology has a corollary, this corollary is rarely presented as such. Indeed, although it is necessary to ensure that a number of signs are present to establish with certainty that a child has ADHD, it should logically be just as necessary to describe the behavioral norm that allows pediatricians to declare that a child does not suffer from it. The question that arises is what model of "child with behavioral tendencies" should be referred to. Once this model has been officially described on the basis of objective criteria (such as school results, forms completed by teachers and degree of commitment to – and success in – school activities), sometimes combined with other more subjective criteria (such as choice of classmates, family situation and siblings, and housing conditions), how can we not assume that there is a drug response for every behavioral deviation of a child? Any behavioral "deficiency" would somehow justify the use of a "corrective" product to cure it. Once explained and corrected as imbalances in the chemistry of neurotransmitters, the disorders induced by these pathologies would no longer disturb the school or the families. As for the child, whose problematic behaviors have been explained to him in terms of neurological disorders, he would only have to take, at a fixed time and in fixed quantities, the medication produced to cure them. For the child and his parents, the endless questioning about their respective responsibilities would be ignored.

To this admittedly approximate description, one can of course retort that it is above all a speculative and polemical – if not outrageously exaggerated – vision. Some will add that it ignores the reality that teachers and relatives are confronted with every day: agitated, disobedient, uncontrollable children. In a word, they are insufferable. As for the potential dangers to which these products could expose these children, one can of course consider that they are exaggerated or even dramatized. Apart from the causes of over-diagnosis which artificially increase the number of cases (Whitely et al., 2019), the medicalization of these children's behavioral disorders has been regularly denounced for years, in Europe as well as in the United States (Landman, 2015; Schwarz, 2016; Saul, 2014).

In this recurrent debate, what happens to the search for the meaning of the child's symptoms advocated by Melanie Klein (2013) in the field of psychoanalysis? At best, the supporters of the medico-scientific approach consider the psychoanalytical approach either useless or merely complementary to a medical treatment. At worst, they are strongly opposed to it and consider that drawing the patient's attention to the content and meaning of his symptoms amounts to diverting him from the rational (and neurological) explanation of the symptoms in question. Indeed, the argument put forward by certain supporters of a strictly neurological etiology of mental disorders is that it is "dangerous" for the patient to be drawn towards a search for the meaning of his symptoms. They claim that science is sufficient to prove that the content of the symptoms has no identifiable rationality.

I will present the case of six-year-old Jordy C., not to demonstrate the harmful effects of the "hard" approach via drug treatment, nor to prove that the psychoanalytical approach is right, but rather to enlighten the debate by taking a position on both the theoretical and clinical levels. To achieve this, it is necessary to give priority to an individual subject and his history and to place the general point of view in the background, thus allowing the "unexpected" to emerge without even attempting to control the symptom, no matter how rationally.

3.   The unique subject and his history

It is now commonplace for teachers faced with a child experiencing academic difficulties to diagnose ADHD on their own initiative. Believing that it is their job to do so, they then ask the child's parents to have the diagnosis confirmed through a medical-psychological intervention. These teachers sometimes mention the possibility of a medical treatment for the child.

3.1.   Jordy's family

It is in such a context that I first saw this six-year-old boy in my office, accompanied by his parents and his brother Kevin.

More than anything, Mr. and Mrs. C. wanted their son to succeed at school, but they also added that they wished to see him stop acting like a baby at home. They said that he was uncontrollable at school. He could not sit still, and according to the teacher, he suffered from a pathological inability to concentrate. The parents both confirmed that at home, he did not obey any more than at school and acted as if he could not hear anything. They also said that he disturbed their intimacy by barging into their bedroom on Sundays, the only day of the week when they could have some peace and quiet. When the mother complained that her son had nighttime anxieties while obstinately refusing to tell her about his dreams, the father pointed out with a half-smile that he himself was the youngest of three boys and that his son was a lot like him when he was a child.

It was clear by the end of the session that since Jordy was the eldest of the three boys, his parents feared he could set a bad example for his two brothers. However, before starting any medical treatment, they agreed to seek the advice of a psychologist. At the end of this first interview, Jordy was eager to come back and meet with me alone. There would be five sessions in all, spaced two weeks apart.

3.2.   Sessions with Jordy

During the first of these sessions, as if he were continuing the exchange he had started with his parents the week before, Jordy started to talk about his difficulties at school without any prompting from me, telling me that he was going to list them to me one subject at a time.

Beginning with his difficulties in math, he said to me: "There is one thing I don't understand how to do, and that is the fill-in-the-blanks exercises."

Jordy was happy to talk and I rarely interrupted him, but I tried to find out if his difficulty lay in understanding the exercise. By way of an answer, Jordy described in detail the instructions given by the teacher and, while maintaining that he could not understand anything, finally concluded, "I get it wrong all the time."

He then went on to speak about his French classes and said: "What I can't do is the exercises where you have to find the odd word out."

As with math, I asked him about his understanding of these exercises. He gave me an example suggesting that it was not a comprehension problem for him and concluded as if stating the obvious: "With odd-words-out exercises, I can't do it."

Instead of continuing to list his difficulties by subject, he began to complain about the teacher's attitude, and summed up what he meant by saying that she was too strict. "Strict?" I said, to which he answered: "At home, my mother is strict too when I'm being stupid."

Intrigued, I asked him what he meant by "being stupid". He did not go into great detail. He just said that it was what he did to his brothers that his mother did not like.

He then sat down in front of the paper and markers that had been there from the beginning of the session and which I had explained he could use to express what he wanted to say when he could not find the words. While drawing his picture, he explained that it was a monster. He added arms to it, one of which was holding a knife. When I asked him about this monster, he told me that it resembled those he saw at night, in his nightmares. He added: "This is for Pascal, isn't your name Pascal? How do you spell it?" (He started to spell it while writing it at the bottom of the sheet.) Then, handing it to me, he said: "He doesn't look very nice. He is sharp, like a mountain." This comparison reminded him of the mountains where he went skiing with his family during the Christmas vacations and he suddenly exclaimed: "Oh, I forgot!" And, taking back his drawing to complete it, he explained to me as he drew that he had forgotten to add a little man with some blood on him and a hole in his belly.

Assuming that this ill-fated little man had an unconscious role in his psychological life, I asked Jordy who the man was. Without hesitation, he answered "It's Yvan," his youngest brother. Then, supposing that this was a murder fantasy, I asked him: "Is the monster you, then?" He reacted immediately: "If I kill him,

I'll be punished! And even if he's dead, I'll still think about him for the rest of my life. But he gets on my nerves!" He then told me in detail about his brother's strategies to "get on his nerves", most often with total impunity, and made the connection with what his parents had said on this subject during the previous session.

Clearly satisfied with this first session, Jordy expressed five times in a row his wish to come back. He concluded our fifth and final meeting by saying: "I don't have nightmares anymore! No more monsters! Now I just have dreams!"

4. Epilogue

Was Jordy, the turbulent or hyperactive child, tormented by nightmares that interfered with his school performance? Could a mere five sessions spent listening to his fantasy life really be enough to put an end to this problem? We need to be humble here. How can one boast of a success which occurred totally unbeknownst to its main witness, and which turned out to be a success only after the fact?

Jordy's father made an appointment a few weeks after his son had completed the treatment. He wanted to talk about himself, since talking had been so successful for his son. During this first interview, which focused on his marital difficulties, a slip of the tongue occurred in which, in his speech, his mother took the place of his wife. Through a long association of ideas, Mr. C. ended up talking about his main reason for concern: the premature ejaculation he was experiencing and which, according to him, could be the cause of his wife's infidelity. Resorting to a far-fetched theory, he tried in vain to alleviate his concern: born by caesarean section, Mr. C. had – so he said – been sexually deprived at his birth of the sensation of passing through the vagina, thus condemning him to premature ejaculation. Concerned about this aspect of his married life, Jordy's father insisted on coming for several months to talk about how sound this theory was, wavering between the love he felt for his wife and the hatred that her infidelity had aroused in him. These sessions came to an end when the school vacation started.

The son's agitation, which had initially incited the family to ask for a consultation, gave the impression of having been in some way passed down by the father to his son. Not only did the father immediately establish a similarity between his son's agitation and his own behavior as a child, but also, once his son was reassured about himself, he in turn wished to be enlightened about his own agitation, which he said he had no control over. Jordy's psychosexual identity continued to be constructed in a relational dynamic in which the father's place seemed insecure and his sexual power uncertain. The Sunday morning games in the marital bed contributed as much to the son's over-excitement as to the father's feeling of powerlessness. The mother's complaints on this subject were undoubtedly linked as much to an unconscious oedipal dimension as to the guilt generated by her extramarital satisfactions, which her husband and her son might have guessed at. In any case, the urges at play in all of them can hardly be separated from the analysis of the symptom, the "official" cause of the parents' decision to consult.

Confusion, turmoil and upheaval occur when the subjective worlds of adults and children meet. It is necessary, however, to distinguish one from the other. Thus, during his sessions, Jordy's father, after having spoken of how his mother would bite him as a child in order to punish him, was astonished to discover that in his mind, and in reality, his wife's bites had taken their place, to be followed in turn by affectionate bites made to Jordy with the sole aim of making him discover "the thrill of pleasure".

Although Ferenczi questioned Freud's teaching, he described the challenge of psychoanalytical work in these terms: "Analysis wins a victory when it succeeds in replacing action by recollection […], the thinking process" (Ferenczi, 1980). In the age of ADHD, which assigns a standardized behavior to the child and authorizes the adult to demand unfailing control of him, it is worth remembering that as early as 1932, Freud's most assiduous pupil remarked how much damage the irruption of adult passion into the subjective universe of the child could cause, most often invisibly. His main recommendation was that:

> parents and adults should learn to recognize, […] behind transference love – the submission or adoration of our children […] –, the nostalgic longing for freedom from this oppressive love. If we help the child […] to abandon this identification, we can say that we have succeeded in bringing the personality to a higher level.
>
> (Ferenczi, 1982).

5. Conclusion

In the future, the so-called "hyperactive" child will undoubtedly have an increasingly important place in general practice consultations. The generalization of the DSM will probably contribute to this, as well as the prospect of a quick and easy-to-implement solution based on medication. While Wallon's psychology announced the importance of an in-depth study of the person-to-person dialogue that is established between the child and the people around him, notably from the dynamic exchanges that take place, psychoanalysis has restored to the content of this research its phantasmatic and libidinal dimension. As for the dynamics of urge at play in the exchanges between adults and children, they are gradually becoming clearer. Can we reduce the dichotomy between the partisans of organicism and psychoanalysts to an opposition between supporters of the hard sciences and those of the soft sciences? Children undoubtedly deserve better than this sterile debate. In any case, theirs is a cause that requires creativity on all sides in order to render obsolete all forms of inertia that are founded on certainties based on sheer belief.

References

Ferenczi, S. (1980). Analyse d'enfants avec des adultes (1980). *Le Coq-Héron*, (75), 5–21.

Ferenczi, S. (1982). Confusion de langue entre les adultes et l'enfant. Le langage de la tendresse et de la passion. In *Psychanalyse 4, Œuvres complètes*, vol. IV: *1927–1933* (pp. 125–135). Paris: Payot.

Klein, M. (2013). *La psychanalyse des enfants*. Paris: Presses Universitaires de France.

Landman, P. (2015). *Tous hyperactifs?* Paris: Albin Michel.

Saul, R. (2014). *ADHD Does Not Exist: The Truth about Attention Deficit and Hyperactivity Disorder*. London: Harper Collins.

Schwarz, A. (2016). *ADHD Nation: Children, Doctors, Big Pharma, and the Making of an American Epidemic*. New York: Simon and Schuster.

Strohl, M. P. (2011). Bradley's Benzedrine studies on children with behavioral disorders. *The Yale Journal of Biology and Medicine, 84*(1), 27–33.

Wallon, H. (1984). *L'enfant turbulent*. Paris: Presses Universitaires de France.

Whitely, M., Raven, M., Timimi, S., Jureidini, J., Phillimore, J., & Landman, P. (2019). Attention deficit hyperactivity disorder late birthdate effect common in both high and low prescribing international jurisdictions: A systematic review. *The Journal of Child Psychology and Psychiatry, 60*(4), 380–391.

Chapter 5

ADHD: from disorder to individual invention

David Coto

***

1. Always more, always faster

"I zapped" and "I zapped you" have become commonplace expressions in colloquial French. The verb *zap* is used to mean that one has forgotten something or someone, that one is engaged in something else or that something else has caught one's attention. It means that one's attention has been diverted to another object.

Zapping thus means letting yourself get caught up in something different from what you were initially paying attention to. It is like switching from one television program to another. It is like that moment when, changing channels during the commercials that interrupt your program, you let yourself become interested in another program, forgetting what you had been watching. *Zapping* means putting everything on the same level and thus smoothly moving from one thing to another. What is at stake here is not only memory; it is also one's capacity for attention as well as the plethora of what is available to us. This capacity for attention diffracts and focuses on everything at the same time.

The term *zap* is derived from the term *zapping* (French for *channel-surfing*), which goes hand in hand with advertising. It thus finds its sources in television and refers to a particular way of watching it. It has become a program in its own right, a montage of heterogeneous sequences, giving the impression of taking everything in all at once: "Did you miss something? Then tune in to the *zapping*!" Today, this term has gone beyond the audiovisual field and designates what could be described as a contemporary symptom: the multiplicity of objects rifled through in a short period of time, the quick passage from one object to another or from one idea to another, instability, a diffracted and ephemeral attention span, incessant movement, agitation, or even hyperactivity. It is a symptom of our modern societies, which are based on excessive consumption and instant gratification.

Zapping thus allows us to consume as much as possible in as little time as possible. It optimizes consumption by inciting people to constantly acquire "new" objects that promise to satisfy their purchaser. Though presented as new, the object

DOI: 10.4324/9781003584469-6

is never anything other than the one you have always been running after, what Lacan calls object *a*. But this is the very principle of consumerism: the so-called "new" object keeps the race going while satisfying nothing, except the race itself. Promise and disappointment, perpetually renewed, drive consumption. This frenzy affects all areas of life. We now speak of romantic *zapping*, ideological *zapping* and tourist *zapping*, for example. Take, for instance, the type of organized trip whose aim is to see as much as possible as quickly as possible. Tourists, trapped in these tours, stop for selfies in front of monuments. The picture is captured and digitized, then immediately posted on social networks, yet another image added to thousands of others to be commented on, pending the next post. Or take online dating sites, where everyone becomes someone else's object of consumption, chosen from a catalogue of filtered images and profiles. With romantic *zapping*, love – or at least what passes for love – gives way to enjoyment, "leading one to dispense [...] with constraints, ideals and commitments" (Deltombe, 2005–2006, p. 34). *Zapping* allows for unfettered and immediate enjoyment. It is an endless slippage that carries away the subjects themselves: they become reduced to being the objects of the objects they consume. Currently, the term *zapping* is in the process of being zapped in turn by another term: *speed* as in *speed dating*, or the new audiovisual phenomenon, *speed watching*, which means watching a television series at a higher speed than normal.

2.   Unlimited access and jouissance

Internet access is now unlimited. Limited-time deals are a thing of the past: providers no longer cut users off. Cuts are to be found elsewhere.

> For the (increasingly low) price of a computer, or even just a mobile phone and an internet connection, billions of humans will soon be able to have access to millions of books, images, songs, films and TV series for next to nothing.
>
> (Citton, 2014, p. 18).

Thus, a lifetime would not be enough to browse through the mass of digital data that makes up the Internet. Many of the teenagers I meet are caught up in this boundless web, much to the dismay of their families. On the web, users do not *zap*, they surf. The metaphor is apt: surfing means staying on the surface as opposed to diving into the depths. We stay on the surface of things and are satisfied with the immediacy of what is seen or heard, no more no less. The more concise the content, the better. A recent trend has teenagers spending less time in front of the television and more on the Internet and smartphones.[1] They surf from one social network, audiovisual platform or content source to another. This is the new form of *zapping*. The overabundant content on offer also exerts an extraordinary force of attraction. We can sometimes get trapped in it when, having to do a search for something specific, we get caught up in the diversity of content and forget what we had originally set out to find. The initial object gets lost, drowned out by the hundreds of others on the screen. Many teenagers find themselves caught up in this vicious circle, in which clicking on one video, for example, brings up dozens of others. The search thus becomes unlimited: clicking on one of them once again leads to a vertiginous labyrinth of more content. One teenager told me he was "lost" on a video content platform. This was his weekend activity, which he described with a certain pleasure. Switching from one video to another, he would find himself lost, absorbing it all and yet unable to exercise judgement. His surfing was like other people's wandering the streets. One might call this "digital wandering." Another teenager interviewed would watch videos to the point of exhaustion. An addiction emerges, and neither the clock nor parental orders can help. And still others are not even aware of their excessive use of the Internet. They surf according to the algorithms that target the content most likely to trigger another click of the mouse or tap of the finger. Thus, the Free Culture (free and unlimited) is linked to the excessive nature of teenagers. The various types of content follow one another at a frantic pace and are sometimes superimposed through the simultaneous use of several screens. The capacity for attention, captured as it is by multiple heterogeneous sources, becomes fragmented. This could be called "digital hyperactivity."

3.   ADHD: between jouissance of the body and the demand of the Other

Attention disorders, hyperactivity and impulsivity thus make up a triptych that goes hand in hand with our consumer society based on a type of *jouissance* that is immediate and unlimited. On the fringes of this modern symptom, of this ambient hyperactivity, we meet children and adolescents diagnosed with "ADHD" whose disorders are so intense that they radically interfere with their social life and academic performance. In a so-called "special education" institution, we see and accompany a good number of children and adolescents who have some or all of the behavioral manifestations described by the term ADHD. It is impossible for them to carry out an activity; they are unable to sit still or concentrate for more than a few minutes; they interrupt and make uncalled-for remarks; they feel an imperious need to be the first to enter or leave the classroom; and they are always losing their personal belongings. These young surfers or zappers of everyday life, whose bodies are in perpetual motion, slip under tables and sneak in and out of rooms. They are unable to deal with the slightest frustration or annoyance. It is in the encounter with the Other at school – that one place where demands are perhaps most explicitly formulated – that these symptoms express themselves most vividly. It is through this encounter that parents are first alerted to their child's symptoms. Faced with various requests, with their teachers' attempts to impart knowledge, the child seems to shrink away, unable to respond adequately to these requests and caught up in all the stimuli that compete with the words and requests of adults. Thus, what agitates these children's bodies seems to take precedence over the words that are addressed to them to such an extent that they seem deaf to them. At other times, they deliver a radical and sharp retort, an attempt to subjectify what escapes them: "I'll do what

I want." The adult's request, whether explicit or implicit, thus remains unheard or thwarted: the child does not respond in the affirmative. To paraphrase Philippe Lacadée, this could well be the signs of an era characterized by Lacan's object *a* having become the individual compass of each *parlêtre* (that is, Lacan's *speaking-being*). This relegates the knowledge of the Other, which carries little weight in the face of the immediate sensations that push each person – in the name of what agitates him – to orient himself more according to his being of *jouissance* than according to the Other of knowledge (Lacadée, 2012, p. 14). In other words:

> Where there were once the ideals impossible for the subject to bear, there is now the body and its *jouissance* in excess, impossible for the Other – parents, teachers, educators – to bear. The problem is complicated by the fact that the Other himself, in his incarnations, is infiltrated by these manifestations of *jouissance* in excess.
>
> (Roy, 2015, p. 10).

Pierre is ten years old. He is one of those children who cannot sit still in the classroom or at the table during meals. His maximum attention span is five minutes. He is in perpetual motion. He spends his time evading the implicit or explicit demands made of him. He is most often detached from the Other, especially from the Other at school, and thus sometimes wanders in the park of the institution where he is being treated, when he should be in class. When I first saw him, it was often impossible for him to stay in my office. He wanted us to go out. We therefore conducted the sessions outside; we walked. He collected leaves, pebbles and branches and put them in a box and started building a hut. The box and the hut were his own private anchors. Pierre then became very bossy and authoritative. He used the imperative when addressing me, telling me what direction to take, the type of stones to find or the branches to collect for his hut. He left little or no room for me to speak. He then gave me a series of orders. He also grabbed a vehicle and loaded it with objects that he held together with a piece of string. This was another form of anchor. He described it as a removal van. Loaded with scattered objects, in perpetual motion and detached from the Other, was this object not an attempt for Pierre to exist in the field of the Other?

Twelve-year-old Sébastien could not stay still either; his attention was extremely scattered. When he entered the office, he would sometimes pounce on anything he saw and ask to use it, only to discard it immediately, as if he were attracted and summoned by each object that crossed his field of vision. This deluge of signifying temptations was interrupted on one occasion, when Sébastien looked at the images of mobile phones found on the Internet and displayed on the computer screen. He stopped moving and wandering around. He selected images to print and paste on cardboard. I then became for Sébastien an instrument, a tool that carried out his orders to build the desired object. Sébastien did not use interrogative formulas to ask whether I consented to what he was asking, let alone polite formulas. Sébastien demanded. He was extremely bossy, even authoritative.

Pierre and Sébastien, each in his own way, were expressing the relationship they had with the demand of the Other. It was an implacable demand that threatened and negated them as subjects, just as they negated me when they addressed me. No verbal language was possible for them in their relationship to the Other, and none was possible for me, crushed as I was by their demands. Do they not show us to what extent they are, as Daniel and Maryse Roy put it, subjects under constraint, for whom any request takes on the value of a command, testifying to an extreme submission to the Other of the request, who becomes a *jouisseur* (Roy & Roy, 2004, p. 34)? In so doing, it is as if they were called upon to respond to all the solicitations of the signifier and, at the same time, to defend themselves from the incessant assaults of the signifying machine (Roy & Roy, 2004, p. 34). Each signifier that comes up exerts an extraordinary force of attraction and demands a response. The subject is thus assailed by heterogeneous signifiers that all have the same weight for him. No hierarchy is possible; the child or adolescent is summoned by each of them and must respond to them, "which leaves him without respite, disturbs [his] attention and agitates [his] body" (Roy & Roy, 2004, p. 34).

4. Deconstructing the category ADHD and extracting from it a subject at work

Our era is thus more interested in what is manifest than what is latent. The famous "black box" located between the stimulus and the behavioral response of a subject is perfectly suited to our era of generalized *zapping* and *speed*. This is not a time for probing the subject's psyche, his fantasies, his representations, his affects, his history or his unconscious, but rather for observing his behavior alone. The symptoms of children and adolescents, as noisy as they are complex, are no exception to this tendency. Each of the young people seen in specialized institutions is presented or presents himself with a number of significant diagnoses that label him too rashly. Profiles of children or adolescents thus emerge from a set of disorders or dysfunctions. In this field, ADHD is at the top of the list. The young people profiled in this way form apparently homogeneous categories, with the same profile calling for the same intervention. However, when these disorders are carefully examined, it becomes obvious that they always turn out to be part of a different history and logic. Thus, although the vast majority of children or adolescents in our institutions show signs of hyperactivity, impulsivity or attentional disorders, or can even be diagnosed with ADHD, this apparent homogeneity does not withstand the scrutiny of those willing to go beyond what can be seen and heard. There emerges a unique subject making a relentless effort to deal with what imposes itself on him in terms of his relationship with his body, with others and with language.

5. Baptiste: finding a voice for what the body imposes

Baptiste was 15 years old when I first saw him. His life had been punctuated by a series of crises and acts of violence. His agitation, impulsiveness and inability to concentrate on his schoolwork were at the forefront of his clinical description.

Baptiste was a young person who could never stay put. His parents said that as soon as Baptiste woke up, which could be very early in the morning, he set about doing household chores. Although engaged in a multitude of activities, he was unable to complete any of them. His parents said that school was difficult from the start. Baptiste was quickly reluctant to consent to the knowledge of the Other.

5.1. Hyperactivity as a treatment?

Baptiste arrived running at the weekly sessions with me. I could hear him from afar, and he would always arrive out of breath, complaining of a stitch in his side. He always seemed to be in a hurry. I understood right away that he could not help himself and was actively trying to slow down the pace at which he moved from one place to another. He would unsuccessfully look for places to stop and for ways to slow down his pace. For example, one day when Christmas was being celebrated in the institution, I saw him arrive all dressed up. He told me that his brand-new shoes would keep him from running because he did not want to damage them, but I could hear him running away as soon as he left my office. Baptiste was driven by a force that pushed him to run constantly. It was like a relentless urge that imposed itself on him and that he could not explain in spite of his efforts to curb it. One of the ways he had found to escape this urge was through movement – a ceaseless movement, a race against time, an endless rush. Baptiste presented a clinical profile that "emphasizes the body as a pure urge-driven object [thereby emphasizing] the acephalous nature of the urge, the absence of intentionality and of subjective identity in this perpetual motion" (Cottet, 2012, p. 80).

5.2. Attempts at subjectivation of the impulse and emergence of an edge

Baptiste told me about the cause of his anguish: it was overflow, more specifically, water overflowing from its container. He quickly spotted a system of gutters on the roof of the neighboring house, visible from my office. These gutters acted as a support for him to formulate a question and attempt to give a name to his anguish. How can the last pipe, the one in which the other gutters end their course, manage to channel the water without overflowing? In other words, how can the water contained in a multitude of pipes finish its course, without overflowing, in a single pipe of the same size as those that flow into it? This question came up regularly during our first sessions and expressed a genuine concern on his part. Could this not have been an attempt by Baptiste to metaphorize what was happening in his body? How could he channel this constant urge which, in the past, had led *him* to overflow in social situations? It was an overflow that he seemed to fear at the time I first saw him. Baptiste evoked the desire to "pass out" as if he could thus disconnect himself from his body – his *corps jouissant* – in order to cut himself off from this constant urge, an urge which he seemed to have difficulty finding a satisfactory way out of.

5.3. Giving form to agitation: manual work

The men in his family were described as hard workers. Baptiste seemed to adopt this signifier to describe his hyperactivity. Indeed, Baptiste said he often worked and puttered around the house. He and his parents mentioned no other activity. There was no time for fun. All Baptiste did was work. Baptiste and I thus came to the conclusion that there seemed to be a need for him to have activities that engaged his body. There had to be movement. From then on, he could engage in an activity in a more lasting way, which was impossible for him when it came to school work, for example. He qualified his agitation as "work". On weekends, for example, he sometimes woke up at four in the morning and brought in some wood. We tried to organize his work at home with his parents. A schedule was devised to limit his *jouissance*. The purpose of this was not to keep Baptiste from working but to divide his days into time slots. This signifier ("work") was also used to offer Baptiste manual tasks at the institution, notably on days when his body was not trapped within a strict timetable. This was the case on Wednesdays, when there were no workshops or classes. These days were particularly difficult for him.

5.4. A new attempt at metaphorization: the car

The work described by Baptiste revolved primarily around housework. He did this at home and would sometimes suddenly pick up a broom in the institution as well, interrupting whatever work he was engaged in. Quite early in the treatment, Baptiste told me about another activity that took up so much of his time that it was now practically all he did: tinkering with old cars. Here again, this was a signifier that was commonly used in his family. Baptiste wanted to share with me his specific knowledge in this field. His sentences were punctuated by the phrase "you know…" when he wanted to show me some model of car on the Internet.

He restored old vehicles and showed them at exhibitions. I came to understand how important these events were for Baptiste: they gave him access to a new temporal dimension. The date of each of these exhibitions punctuated his work, allowing for a discontinuity, whereas household tasks were part of a continual flow. Indeed, the vehicles on display had to be ready on the scheduled dates. These deadlines allowed Baptiste to enter into a new relationship with time, the idea that you have to be ready on time, that is to say, you have to finish what you have been working on, but above all you have to wait for the date. Baptiste seemed to be very sensitive to this new organization of time. We talked about the weekend's schedule and the order in which the vehicles had to be repaired. Through this symbolic imaginary material – that is, the cars – Baptiste was able to engage in a new attempt to deal with part of what was imposed on him. It was a new metaphorical way to channel the urge and to attempt to make it socially acceptable, an edge or boundary (*bord*, in French) allowing him to give form to his movements and to sublimate his agitation. Two expressions allowed him to express his difficulty and also his attempt at finding a solution: "revving up the engine" referred to his agitation, his urge to act and his impulsiveness; "braking" referred to the attempt to channel the engine's surge, the excess and the overflow. Thus, Baptiste tried to name the urge and to channel it. These metaphors, borrowed from the field of mechanics, served as an attempt to pin down what acts within the body. Baptiste started telling me that he was "braking with his shoes", but that from time to time he had to "change the brake pads". The weekly sessions seemed to become his brake pad "maintenance" workshop, a time-space where we listened to his ways of naming what agitated him and what made it possible to lower the engine speed, to slow down the race and the panic – a place where action and haste made way for speech. I noted then that Baptiste yawned a lot during the interviews. He complained of intense fatigue. He began slowing down.

5.5. A turning point, a real: love at first sight as a new way out of the urge?

One day during a session, Baptiste wanted to tell me about an encounter with a friend. It was an encounter that had moved him deeply. He described a case of love at first sight the moment he saw a boy who was "running around". Baptiste explained to me that he was overwhelmed by the image of this young man, whose face appeared to him, jumped out at him, as it were. It imposed itself on him. He could not manage to shake it off. He said he was in love, and yet this friend aroused in him a great deal of violence: he felt like fighting, he said. Baptiste explained that he could not stop; what had been imposing itself on him was now out in the open. The urge possessing him had now taken an actual shape, that of the friend towards whom he could not help but go or imagine himself going. It was a movement focused entirely on this new object, which had become exclusive. This was a high-risk period for Baptiste, who felt he was on the verge of acting out.

5.6. The invention of two boundaries?

Musical apparatus

Cars, and working on cars, had become an important part of Baptiste's treatment. This object allowed him to occupy a position of knowledge. His saying "you know" to me allowed him not only to create a social link but also to change my position. It was undoubtedly at this price that Baptiste could continue with the work I proposed to him. I was put in the position of a pupil, a learner. In this way, he distanced himself from the knowledge of the Other. Another theme quickly emerged in Baptiste's discourse around the phrase "you know…". This object was music. Baptiste had equipped himself with a device for playing music. From then on, the two objects – music and cars – became connected with the phrase "you know…". I could no longer hear Baptiste constantly running, but I could hear the music he was now listening to very loudly. "I take this thing with me wherever I go," he said of his device. I gave this object its due value: a treatment-object, a personal invention that obviously helped Baptiste to keep at bay what was imposed on him. We noted how much he needed to detach himself from that nameless urge. This was what music enabled him to do, music and also working on cars. He explained to me that music was becoming the object that helped him to fall asleep quickly, whereas before he had found this so difficult. He also explained that when he woke up very early, he either worked or listened to music. The music allowed him to postpone movement. We talked about the rhythm of the music. Baptiste explained to me that he liked music with a fast rhythm but that sometimes he could adjust and slow down the rhythm with his MP3 player. He set it to the minimum. The music and its rhythm, which he tuned into, seemed to impose a slightly slower tempo on him, which calmed him down. The device and the music it played were becoming an extension of his own body, which regulated what the body imposed.

A new term serving as a "brake": teenager

The music from the device allowed Baptiste to delay the onset of his urge to move, but it was also an object which many teenagers equip themselves with and use wherever they go. Many of them have such a device in their hand or pocket. Baptiste seemed to have adopted this fashion accessory, one that teenagers carry around as they would wear a piece of clothing. This commonly shared signifier was part of a new identification: that of "teenager". Thus, after complaining of pains following a race, Baptiste said to me: "I used to run, but I don't anymore […]. I act like a teenager […]. And teenagers are lazy." Baptiste identified with the "teenager" and adopted certain traits such as nonchalance or sleeping late in the morning. If, when experiencing love at first sight, Baptiste could demonstrate a kind of mirror relationship with the other in whom he recognized himself, could this not be a form of "imaginary stabilization" (Stevens, 2018, p. 6-64) that does not rely on "the Other of the symbolic, but the little other […], which is often observed in certain psychotic subjects and gives a strict mode of identification" (Borie, 2012, p. 75)? Following the viewing of a clip where sexual desire was coupled with the topic of cars, Baptiste said he felt less overwhelmed and could control himself better.

6.   Léo is hyperactive: but what else?

Léo was 14 years old when I first saw him at a therapeutic workshop. From the start, he appeared as an extremely agitated child. He ran, jumped, screamed, pushed others, threw himself on the floor and climbed on the furniture. When part of a smaller group, he was calmer and clung to adults. Léo was diagnosed as "hyperactive"; he took medication to treat this disorder but it had never improved his behavior. His agitation had even increased to the point where it had become temporarily impossible for Léo to continue living in a community setting. His whole behavior – his hand in his pants, his *love you*'s, his incessant embraces – testified to an experience of reality that suddenly seemed to invade his body. Faced with the tidal wave of puberty, Léo could no longer control anything.

6.1. Leaping and bouncing to feel alive?

Léo was constantly agitated. He was always running. You could hear him coming from afar. He would slam doors to get where he wanted to go, sometimes ignoring the obstacles in front of him. Léo was said to "bounce off" the walls and other people's bodies. These were the only objects that seemed to border the infinite, unsymbolized world in which he seemed to live. Only three moments in the day slowed him down, three times which structured his daily life. Meals were a sacred moment; they stopped his incessant movements, but the overflow continued. He would gobble up his meal, and the staff had to limit the quantities of food. Otherwise Léo would not stop eating. Another occasion when he would stop bouncing about was when music was playing. The agitation would take another form. He would begin to sway. His movements then were unusually intense and precise at the same time. Léo just grazed the wall with the back of his head, never bumping into it. The pool was also an important time, a moment of respite for him and his caregivers. The water utterly enveloped him. They said how much he seemed to be fighting against tiredness, how he seemed not to be able to let go. Only when he was alone in a room could Léo finally settle down and often fall asleep. Once he was cut off from the Other, his agitation seemed to give way at last. Sheltered from the stimuli that assailed him and forced him to respond, Léo could find some peace.

6.2. Working on the edge

When Léo arrived at the institution, he had to sit between two adults when eating. Otherwise, it was impossible for him to have a quiet meal. He could not sit still and would slip under the table. In the workshop sessions, I noticed that Léo was constantly trying to get into corners, be it the corner formed by the junction of two walls, one of the corners formed by the partitions of the office or the corner of a shelf. Léo got into corners, and that stopped him. Over the course of the sessions, Léo was able to stay away from corners and lean against a wall. At that time, he would use small objects – such as cars, figurines and even fences – to surround himself with. He started to build the edges that contained him. He would find himself sitting in the middle of a square formed on three sides by the rows of objects, with the wall forming the fourth side. The perimeter thus drawn was off-limits to others. Léo found this soothing. The juxtaposed objects seemed to form an edge and allowed him to remain in the group. Thus protected, keeping the Other at a distance, he could consent to a few other people interacting with him but on his own terms. Léo took great care building this edge. In the institution, he always took the same route. When walking, he kept close to the walls of the buildings, choosing to take the sometimes narrow paths around the houses.

6.3. Where there is no body, there is agitation

It was not uncommon for Léo to forget to put on his shoes to go out, or a coat when the temperatures required it. In sports, Léo's performance was impressive.

He could run at the same pace and never slow his speed. He did not seem to feel the physiological limits of his body. During several sessions in the workshop, Léo asked me to make him some accessories for his body such as cardboard watches, bracelets or crowns. I came to understand his need for these objects to hold him tight. Léo left the sessions thus adorned with cardboard, surrounding his head or his wrists. Jacques-Alain Miller points out that the "schizophrenic patient [...] has the feeling of being outside his body, and he has to invent, as he says, devices to bind himself to his body" (Miller, 2004, p. 5). He explains what these devices are in the case of a man he is describing:

> He puts rings on his fingers to bind them to his body. On his head, he puts a band to bind it to the body. [...]. These are attachments that are put on organs, parts of the body.
>
> (Miller, 2004, p. 5).

Miller adds that in this subject, there was no "I". I was able to hear Léo say "I" on only one occasion. It was a striking moment. He was very agitated and unable to stop moving around the room, so I took one of the many crowns we had made and put it on his head. The next moment, he froze and said: "I am stuck." The crown seemed to unify his fragmented body: Léo was expressing how he felt. The agitation ceased the moment he created his own body. This is where Léo's invention lay, adorning himself with chef's hats, headbands or elastic bands that he would place on his head. It put him in one place, just as he used to try to put himself into corners or between two people.

7. From one real to another

Baptiste and Léo show us that what can be seen and heard is necessary but not sufficient. They invite us to go beyond a clinic of surfaces and of what is manifest, and to dive into the depths of the unconscious and of *jouissance*. Both show signs of great agitation, instability, attention disorders, impulsivity and hyperactivity, but this is part of a logic specific to each one of them – a specific logic which requires a different kind of care. They also demonstrate a process that asserts itself on them and that is the sign of an irrepressible and unspeakable urge that manifests itself in the open. The specific inventions that they devise are the fruits of this psychological process. They act as levers that support their way of coping with that irreducible part of the real each of them must confront.

The real we are talking about here is not that which is hidden in the brain, that is, that real with universalizing and objectifying claims that dispenses with the subject's speech. The real we are talking about is the one that is inherent in the exercise of language and in the way it impacts the *jouissant* body of each One – a body that, by experiencing itself, pierces through the signifying fabric and produces what is impossible to say for each *parlêtre*.

Baptiste and Léo direct us towards this real, a different real for each of them, and each with his own body, each with his own language, each with his own impossibility.

Note

1 https://www.lesechos.fr/tech-medias/medias/television-la-baisse-de-la-duree-decoute
-se-poursuit-1039780

References

Borie, J. (2012). *Le psychotique et le psychanalyste*. Paris: Éditions Michèle.

Citton, Y. (2014). *Pour une écologie de l'attention*. Paris: Éd. du Seuil.

Cottet, S. (2012). *L'inconscient de papa et le nôtre*. Paris: Éditions Michèle.

Deltombe, H. (2005–2006). L'insaisissable désir à l'adolescence. *Les documents de Scripta*. Saint-Quentin: Association de la Cause Freudienne Champagne-Artois-Picardie-Ardennes.

Lacadée, P. (2012). *Vie éprise de parole*. Paris: Éditions Michèle.

Miller, J.-A. (2004). L'invention psychotique. *Quarto*, (80/81), 6–13.

Roy, D. (2015). Énigme et défi. In *Interpréter l'enfant* (pp. 7–12). Paris: Navarin éditeur.

Roy, D., & Roy, M. (2004). Hyperactivité: ordre et désordres. *La Cause Freudienne*, (58), 28–36.

Stevens, A. (2018). *La psychose ordinaire et les stabilisations par l'imaginaire*. Montréal: Le Pont Freudien.

Chapter 6

Anastasia: a new choreography

Laurence Morel

***

1. Introduction

Anastasia's story could be seen as exemplifying the notion that hyperactivity is a cause-and-effect phenomenon. After all, from the day she was born, all odds were against her. One might then imagine that some sound child-rearing would put some order into her chaotic start in life. But I propose to look at things from a different angle and to point out the impact of language on the trajectory of this child, through the encounter between words and the body. In Anastasia's case, analysis became a support point, a space for rewriting her history in an attempt to ground a new desire.

In such cases, what is needed is time. Time, indeed, but also chance encounters that can turn out to be instances of *bon-heurt*, or blessings in disguise. In the public service sector, where reducing waiting times is a genuine concern, the temptation is strong to prescribe short psychotherapies, in which the symptom and the suffering are ignored in favor of a management approach aimed at eradicating the disorders.

Yet, in a way, a symptom can be beneficial to a child. It allows a child to address an Other who tries to hear her, to follow her step by step in order to "loosen the stranglehold" (Miller, 2001) in which her being is caught, whatever may be the early identifications and obstacles she encounters as she matures.

Freud recognized the symptom's "function as a defense against the traumatic experience of sexuality and as an escape from anxiety" (Roy, 2021).

2. The child and her symptoms: agitation and anxiety

When a distraught Mrs. B. called to ask for her two-and-a-half-year-old daughter to be seen in the institution where I worked, I could hear the child screaming in the background, demanding to take the telephone from her mother. I made an appointment for both of them. At that first meeting, the mother went straight to the point: "Whenever she comes back from her father's house, she's hysterical. It all started

DOI: 10.4324/9781003584469-7

the first time she went there without me. She doesn't listen to anyone. She screams, and so I scream too, and she cries. Do whatever it takes to get her to sleep again. She can't function properly!"

This mother's interpretation was that her daughter was purposely doing everything she could to infuriate her mother and make her scream from morning to night. I recognized in these two individuals an instance of the "couple formed by a dynamite-child and an exacerbated mother" (Cottet, 2012, p. 85).

This little girl's mother explained to me the chaotic life she had experienced with the child's father until the child was one year old. The parents did little more than exchange screams, insults and rants. There was no room, it seems, for what Dominique Laurent calls a "conversation between the parents, or those who fulfill this role with the child, [which] contributes to putting a brake on the unlimited economy of *jouissance*" (Laurent, 2021).

She denounced this man's obscenity and vulgarity towards her – he would tell her, for example, that "all women are sluts". She ultimately felt so persecuted that she left him. On top of that, his two sons had returned to the house and were violent with her during her pregnancy. Anastasia was her father's sixth child and would remain her mother's only child.

The judge ruled that, when the child visited her father, she was to go alone. Mrs. B. was vehemently critical of his alcohol abuse and of the unacceptable living conditions for such a young child. Every time Anastasia came back home, her mother would take her to the emergency room and demand a medical certificate proving that the child's health was being adversely affected. The doctors did not seem alarmed and did not follow up on her requests. An investigation carried out at the father's home revealed no serious negligence.

During a telephone conversation I had with him, the father first said that he suspected the visits to the hospital to be attempts to deprive him of the custody of his daughter. Then, somewhat reassured, he asked me if I was worried about her.

Anastasia had certain recurrent behaviors. She would move from one activity to another without ever settling down. When addressing adults, she would shout and act out her overwhelming agitation in a flow of boundless, erratic episodes. She seemed to act as a mirror to the incessant conflicts between her parents, staging characters and making them scream and fight. Nevertheless, she was surprised to see that I was interested in what she was doing and thus took an interest in our exchanges. Unfortunately, these early visits were interrupted. The mother had health problems and would occasionally forget the appointments. At the same time, Anastasia's father had grown weary of the conflict and would forget to pick up his daughter. Such neglect was to leave its mark on the child.

***

I saw Anastasia again three years later. At five and a half, the slightly chubby little girl I had known a few years earlier was now obese – as her mother had always been – and complained that she could not hear me: "I'm deaf," she cried out at the top of her lungs. It would take time for the mother to react and to consult an ear, nose and throat specialist for her daughter. She had other concerns: maintaining the precarious balance of her daily life, taking care of her house, working with children in difficult circumstances and recovering various objects from the rubbish dump, objects she would then sell to make a little money.

Anastasia rushed to her mother's breasts as she spoke to me, literally hanging on to them while groping them with busy fingers and staring at her with eager eyes. It was as though the words that came out of her mother's mouth were being swallowed up by the girl: she was unable to take her eyes and attention off her mother's body. Later, she said that she insisted on sleeping in her mother's bed to prevent her from taking a lover. Maryse Roy comments on the "attention of these children [referred for hyperactivity] entirely fixated on their mother's libido" (Roy, 2001, p. 69).

Anastasia would pounce on anything she coveted: any object that another person possessed immediately became what she wanted for herself. She immediately sucked in everything within earshot and captured everything in her field of vision. Anastasia was ravenous: she wanted to devour everything. She stuffed herself with every food she could get her hands on, to the frustration of the various dieticians she went to. Anastasia's mother was the first to undermine her daughter's dietary restrictions: "You can't ask a child to make such an effort," she protested.

On two occasions, following an injury, follow-up appointments at the hospital for her obesity were postponed.

With this child, I knew I would have to go slowly and try to avoid any approach that might appear overly interventionist. From then on, I would attempt to harness the boundlessness Anastasia was suffering from.

Nothing could stop this little girl, in her body and in her words. She called out to anyone in her field of vision as though mesmerized and carried away by never-ending agitation. This was evidenced by the spirals she scribbled excitedly during the sessions.

She expressed herself using a rich and precise vocabulary and occasionally expressed her fear of the "mean brother" her father hit with a dishcloth and of the way the man screamed at the boys and at his new wife.

Perturbed by the words that flowed through her, Anastasia would panic and speak out of turn like a weathervane spinning in all directions. She was invaded by the speech of the Other; the words flowed through her but their meanings could not take hold. Her mother's words struck her body, and she became agitated as soon as her mother spoke. What this revealed was the inner disorder that had always agitated her, for lack of an interpretive mechanism that could have pacified her world and organized meaning.

Anastasia talked about what made her suffer and told me about the nightmares that had been haunting her "since I was a baby", or "as long as I've been alive". In one of the nightmares, "a whale with many heads devours everyone". In another, "a very big, strong, slimy monster devours my family, kills them and burns them up. A slimy monster that is still alive when you kill it. And every time it makes babies that then become monsters, too."

Defenseless when dealing with an Other with an unlimited desire for *jouissance*, Anastasia fell prey to terrors that haunted her nights and gave rise to nightmares. A few private conversations with Mrs. B. revealed to me certain elements of her history that resonated with the signifiers that appeared in these nightmares, in particular the "baby-making monster".

A very distressed Anastasia also told me about hallucinations that could arise at any time of the day or night. She could hear a deep voice saying: "the – the – the – the"; "Anastasia … Listen."

The girl was left wondering what it might mean. A "Pssst! pssst!" came out of nowhere and called out to her. In an attempt to banish these voices, Anastasia shook her head when she was alone: "How can I make it stop?" she implored.

Because she was able to talk about it during our sessions, the voices became rarer and lost their intensity. An interesting article by Sonia Chiriaco can help to better understand this effect:

> [When a patient addresses] an Other who agrees to be a recipient, the phenomenon will already appear less threatening. The analyst who is willing to hear this is first and foremost a witness who allows the subject to come out of the radical isolation in which he finds himself. [...] Once translated into words, the voice is no longer pure reality. The symbolic – language – and the imaginary are added to it. [...] The patients suppose that the analyst knows what is interfering with them. This supposition allows them to ask for help. [...] Until then, only the Other as *jouisseur*, the Other whose toy the subject was, was supposed to know, and even to know everything. [...] Thanks to transference, the Other will become fragmented.
>
> (Chiriaco, 2008, p. 25)

Anastasia was completely unfocused. The words used in her presence seemed to pass through her without any filter to protect her from them or to allow her to find shelter. She was assailed by sentences apparently caught on the fly in her daily life, sentences that she mumbled during her games or that arose haphazardly in her conversations.

Her speech was dominated by metonymy. Words tumbled out of her mouth without rhyme or reason. She jumped from one idea to another, constantly changing the subject. I tried to stop her and asked her to take the time to explain any little detail that I did not understand. The sessions then became short breaks in the never-ending whirlwind of her life.

When given pencil and paper, she would draw something with one hand and then, as fast as lightning, erase it with the other. Indefatigably, I stuck to my strategy. I showed interest, congratulated her, expressed my astonishment, commented and asked questions. This surprised her, and she stopped to tell me what she had drawn or what she wanted to redo immediately when not satisfied with her work. Brief moments of silence occurred so that she could find the words to express what she wanted to say. As soon as she became irritated, my patience and careful listening encouraged her. She told me that she liked learning at school and writing. But she was afraid that her mother would stop reading stories to her if she knew about it.

She talked about her mother's systematic refusal to grant her wishes. And, indeed, her mother was quite ready to believe that her daughter wanted to "take her place". Anastasia found it impossible to make herself heard by her mother. The frequent conflicts between herself and her mother inevitably degenerated. Faced with what was assailing her – and with what she sensed as exasperation on the part of her mother – Anastasia declared to her mother: "It would have been better if I hadn't been born!" As pointed out by Jacqueline Dhéret,

> Since there is no answer in the symbolic system to the question "why did you bring me into being", the subject must be accountable for his or her own being, with whatever means are available.
>
> (Dhéret, 2007, p. 78)

These means, which were very precarious for Anastasia, nevertheless gradually became fleshed out as our sessions progressed. Speech allowed her to create footholds that supported her. Although it is up to each child to be able to "adopt his or her origin" (Ansermet, 2021), and although this "also involves being adopted by a desire" (Ansermet, 2021), we will now look at some of the highlights of the desire that led to Anastasia's birth, shaped by both the father's neglect and her mother's difficult past.

3. "A family of wackos"

The conditions surrounding Anastasia's birth are marked by an inexorable cycle in her mother's life, punctuated by the tragedy and unfortunate encounters that would weave the threads of her fate.

Mrs. B. was certain that Anastasia's father wanted to marry her with the sole purpose of getting her pregnant so that he could recover custody of his boys. Had she even wanted a child? That was far from sure. She did want one, but all she could think of was her own father forcing himself on her once his wife could no longer fulfill the role of bearing him children.

An obscene and ferocious *jouissance* became the child's companion, without there being any symbolic link. Christiane Alberti says that "the springboard, the foundation [of the prohibition of incest] is the condition for the world of demand and desire to subsist: in other words, the world of speech as such. The object of incest is forbidden and there is no other object" (Alberti, 2021). As far as her relationship with her own mother went, Mrs. B. had experienced "cruelty". She would even come to regret her father's absence – he died when she was in her early twenties. He would not have let her mother be so cruel to her, she said. The mother, who was obese herself, would make fun of her daughter's size, humiliating and disparaging her. At the age of 8, the child dreamed of becoming a singer and dancer. Her hopes were ruined by her mother, who had always put her down: "You are fat." This irrevocable condemnation seemed to have marked the girl's body and to have permanently trapped her in a degrading image which left no room for the future.

During the years of my sessions with Anastasia, the devastating link between Mrs. B. and her own mother weakened a little when she decided to go to her mother's house less often, thus putting an end to the mockery aimed at both her and her daughter. Aided by the transferential link and my disapproval of the jibes she was complaining about, she started asking herself questions: "But she's the one who fed me! How can she blame me for being fat?" "Indeed," I replied with a knowing wink. "She's been stuffing you with blame, hasn't she? Why don't you stop swallowing *that*?"

Having satisfied her father's incestuous advances and fallen prey to her mother's ferocious *jouissance*, Mrs. B. was left with no other option. At the age of 18, in order to "save herself", she decided to climb out of her bedroom window to escape her hellish homelife, to "free herself from this family of wackos," to borrow the expression that Anastasia would use to express her own situation. But it was only to find herself trapped in another form of hell, in the clutches of a woman who would sequester her for 11 years, making her her slave.

There was no solution to be found through speech, no way to say "no" to the Other, but taking action in order to escape the worst actually worsened her downward slide. This would lead to Anastasia's realization that her mother was capable of the worst: she now feared that the little cat her mother hated so much would be thrown out the window, as had already happened to her things when she had neglected to put them away.

In the relationship with her daughter, a figure of persecution thus reappeared to the mother; it was as though the threat of subservience to an Other was always about to rear its head and force her to be a slave. She complained about her daughter and about being treated like nothing more than her servant. Her childhood experiences and unfortunate encounters had left an indelible mark on her. She could only imagine future misfortune and failure for her daughter. The inertia preventing the emergence of a symptom that could have been beneficial inevitably remained at a complete standstill: "It will always be like this." She could not differentiate her daughter from other people in the family whom she looked after from time to time. Thus, Anastasia did not matter to her any more than any of her nephews: they were all the same to her. This left no room for any particular desire that might have been a sign of love for her daughter.

In the relationship between Mrs. B. and Anastasia, an operator was undoubtedly missing that would allow "a certain distance, an 'inter-diction' between child and mother. [An operator that] can be situated beyond the sexual partner [but that] is a fact of language and allows the child to situate himself or herself as alive and sexualized" (Laurent, 2021).

Anastasia told me that she sometimes wanted to kill herself, to join her grandfather whom she had never known, but nonetheless missed. In the absence of what should have been symbolized, it was a separation in reality that arose, calling her in turn to the radical separation that suicide would be. I told her that there was no one to see on the other side, in order to curb her death wish and to incite her to find another way to reach whatever she desired. I did this by asking her to speak about the things that interested her.

4.   A diabolical couple: mother and child

Failing to find a way to contain her daughter's boundlessness through words, Mrs. B. complained that she had no more room and that her daughter was invading her space, following her everywhere, deciding everything, speaking out of turn, regularly throwing tantrums in the shops she took her to and never putting her things away – she (Mrs. B.) who, in order to position herself with respect to her siblings, had said that she was the "halfway point", that is, halfway between the eldest and the youngest. The only way Mrs. B. could find to deal with her daughter was through violence: she raised her voice, slapped her, and realized that she might one day just keep hitting her and not be able to stop. She said that she was not apt to help her daughter and wondered what use to her she was.

Any attempt to get herself out of this symbiotic, deleterious relationship with her daughter and to find other interests brought her back to the impossibility of separation. Thus, at work – where, for lack of a symbolic anchoring which might otherwise have given her a framework for the position she occupied, she wanted, apparently, "to save all the children" – she found herself having difficulty and losing her balance. She became violent and had to take sick leave on several occasions. She also decided to take up dancing, an activity she had enjoyed when she was younger, but she joined a club near her mother's house, once again coming under her fire.

Anastasia's mother was at her wits' end and was afraid of doing something she would regret. Her daughter's visits to her father's house brought back the nightmare that Mrs. B. had fled from in her youth: "He ruined everything," she kept saying.

By wanting to see his daughter, he broke the routine she had established after she had left the house with her daughter.

Thus, mother and daughter, in a mirror-like relationship, could not separate from each other. Mrs. B. took a job as close as possible to her daughter's school and never took her eyes off her. Their daily life, day and night, became a living hell. Mrs. B. complained that her daughter stole food from her, "treated her like a dog" and wanted to "take her place". Mrs. B. found it alarming that when she slept, Anastasia thought she was dead.

The urge for violence increased, with no possibility of separating mother from daughter. She still feared that she would hit her daughter without being able to stop herself and told social services about it. With great ambivalence, she finally agreed to consider foster care so that something could be done about a relationship in which violence and shouting were now reaching a climax.

When Anastasia was eight years old, it was agreed that she would spend a few days a week away from home. She found this decision intolerable, cried a lot, was inconsolable and regretted having been mean to her mother, thinking that she was being punished for it. Anastasia begged me to intervene and reduce this sentence, promising to be a perfect little girl from then on.

Many of the sessions became the stage on which this unbearable situation could be played out. Listening to Anastasia, I encouraged her to talk to me about what was happening to her and the minor events in her life, which she agreed were not all catastrophic. She acknowledged that her childminder helped her with her lessons and that she was kind. Anastasia learned to establish limits there, which she still could not do at her mother's house. Later on, she would come to see that her mother herself had no limits and she would realize that this painful separation had in fact been beneficial.

5.   Escaping from the mother's grip: from ranting to writing

For a long time, Anastasia had relied on what could be written. At first, "writing" seemed to echo the "ranting" that, in reality, punctuated the chaos of her daily life. However, little by little, writing took shape, bringing some measure of order to her world. She impulsively scribbled on a sheet of paper what she wanted to explain to me, using confused diagrams that I questioned one after the other, assuring her of my ignorance. Then we looked up in the dictionary the insulting words her peers used to humiliate her – they called her "fat". The synonyms, the definitions and the literal or figurative meaning of the words wove a web that gave her the opportunity to somewhat lessen the impact of the insults which she was the target of. When Mrs. B. came to see me, she scrupulously wrote down in her notebook what I suggested "so as not to forget." It was a kind of aid that, although fragile, nevertheless laid down some reminders that she could take home with her after our talks. She knew that she could count on a few other well-meaning people. This sometimes kept her in line and enabled her to reach out. No matter how precarious, it was a safety net that held her back in moments of crisis.

The fairy tales that Anastasia staged during our sessions allowed her to come up with signifiers that had marked her mother's life: the witch and the wicked queen each used their evil powers to get the better of the other and both "wanted it all," casting spells and poisoning innocent victims. Cinderella, held captive, was a slave to her wicked stepmother. Anastasia protested, quoting the definition of the word "slave": "it means working without being paid". She began to build dreams for herself in which she made a lot of money: she would be rich, famous and happy.

Either her nightmares were becoming less frequent or she no longer remembered them. The hallucinations subsided.

Anastasia liked to write. She also liked to sing and had started to write down songs in a notebook her maternal grandmother had given her. But, said the grandmother, "It's to keep her mouth shut," because she hated to hear her granddaughter sing.

Anastasia spoke to me of her grandmother's wickedness and took offense to it. Danger seemed to be looming over her once again. Seeking to protect her from the ferocity of this evil *jouissance* that words only served to increase, we invented a way to laugh about it, euphemistically criticizing her grandmother's "very bad temper". The sessions, for Anastasia, were the place where she worked step by step to de-construct what she was still the target of.

Writing these songs, which she jotted down on slips of paper that she brought to my sessions, kept her very busy and distracted her from the ever-present conflicts in her daily life at home or at school. In her songs, she chose her words carefully. She would sing, proofread, correct, ask my opinion and time herself, mindful of what it meant to post clips on *YouTube*: we could now begin working on establishing limits.

She looked for ways to separate herself from her mother. Having experienced the fundamental refusal of the Other towards her, Anastasia slipped into her songs a discreet "shut the f... up" addressed to her mother – she now knew better than to utter the insult out loud. She told me that she knew that you can't say these things. Both mother and daughter had to deal with the same propensity for impulsive outbursts, and the child learned how to give a form to them. She relied on the Other in order to manage the ranting and to contain it.

Mrs. B. started to periodically complain again, but the targets had now changed from her daughter to her own mother and to her daughter's father, who was reasserting his rights while refusing to pay any more child support. This made Mrs. B. furious.

During these moments of crisis, Anastasia felt sick. She had headaches and bellyaches. She did not want to go to school anymore and referred to "a whirlwind", which she called a "tornado". The nightmares came back, in the guise of a horrible creature who wanted to skin her alive. Voices started haunting her again: "Get into your mother's bed or I'll break your neck!"

Anastasia complained that her father did not love her since he no longer took her to his house. She mentioned again that she wanted to kill herself in order to join her grandfather who, she was sure, would have taken care of her. She said she did not know her grandfather's first name but that she would inquire about it when she was older.

The lack of symbolic transmission through this name that cannot be inscribed left her vulnerable to the temptation of suicide. I encouraged her to write down what she wanted, and so she decided to write a letter to the judge asking both to see her father and to "be protected".

During these sessions, she would come up with problematic scenarios and devise solutions: for example, she imagined a train traveling along clifftops. The track it followed was long and treacherous, so she undertook to build another track.

6.   Inhabiting a body

Anastasia's story shows that having a body is not self-evident. For a subject, the body is elaborated in the relationship with the Other of the signifier. It is not a given from the outset, but is taken up in a construction woven with, on the one hand, the image in the mirror and, on the other hand, the words of the Other that bestow a body on the subject. The small child in front of the mirror, carried and looked at by the Other, apprehends its body as separate from the one who carries it (Lacan, 1966, pp. 93–100). Named, spoken of, it will lodge its being in the desire of the Other. The body, says Lacan, acquires a mental consistency:

> The *parlêtre* adores his body, because he believes that he has it. In reality he does not have it, but his body is his only consistency – a mental consistency, of course, because his body can fall apart at any moment.
>
> (Lacan, 2005, p. 66)

Thus, for the body to exist for a subject, there must be this conjunction of the symbolic order and the dimension of the unified image of the body, which is formed at the mirror stage.

At the age of ten, Anastasia already had the fully developed body of a teenager. She dressed in tight-fitting clothes, doing her best to keep her balance on high heels and wearing the sparkling jewelry a woman would wear.

At each session, Anastasia wedged herself between the seat of the chair and the desk, as if to hem in her body.

> The most intimate disorder is this breach in which the body unravels and where the subject is led to invent artificial ties to reappropriate his body, to "tighten" his body to himself. To put it in mechanical terms, he needs a clamp to hold his body together.
>
> (Miller, 2009, p. 46)

Wedged in and solidly anchored, Anastasia could begin each of her sessions. The eroticization of her body, her desire to seduce and to draw attention to herself, were all delicate subjects. Her mother noticed these transformations when puberty set in and, far from realizing how precarious and worrying all this was, praised this body, which gave her daughter the appearance of a little woman. I took a different view and gently tried to discourage what seemed to me premature for a girl her age. What I encouraged instead had to do with the question of desire.

Anastasia asked her mother about puberty. The crude explanations she received in return did not fail to trigger the most incredible fantasies: for example, on the subject of the onset of menstruation, Anastasia shuddered to think that sharks could come and devour her, attracted by the blood. I told her that she certainly had a lot of imagination, and she laughed.

It was also through the use of objects that Anastasia seemed to give substance to her body, in lieu of a phallic signification that she lacked, to give value to her being. She collected various gadgets that she brought regularly to her sessions. She showed me her treasures: *Star Wars* or *Pokemon* cards she had picked up in supermarkets or exchanged with others. Thanks to these objects, she tried to create a social link that remained precarious, admitting to me that deep down she did not care. But she found that these provided a semblance of connection with others of her age at school. Among these cards, which after all were not very important to her, there were some that she was nevertheless rather fond of, such as the play banknotes that she brought me one day, on the back of which were inscriptions in Japanese.

7.   Choreography: the beginnings of a new meaning

At the dawn of adolescence, and without recourse to the mediation that a father would have provided, how could she bring about separation properly? Between clinging to her mother and violently breaking away, she had to find her own personal path.

Anastasia had been fascinated for some time by the videos she watched on *YouTube*, featuring the bodies of Asian teenagers. The heroes who save young people from danger and the beautiful heroines who sing and dance so brilliantly captivated and attracted her. One day, she would go to this land of dreams, where, far from her mother at last, she would be famous and make her fortune. To do so, she realized that she would have to learn a foreign language. I emphasized how crucial this step would be. This significantly distanced the actualization of a project that over-excited her and created a sense of urgency that was potentially dangerous. For her, the very name of the country was synonymous with the choreography that she loved in these videos and that she tried in her turn to create. Dancing, as a means to sublimate the body, was also what her mother would have liked to do since childhood.

It is a form of writing, then, that ties the body (*corps*, in French) to beautiful forms, a *corps*-and-graphy (or "corps-et-graphie") that, for Anastasia, could be an invention to channel the agitation that overwhelmed her, a way to enclose the body and to make it a vessel for desire as well.

These dreams, which she told me about during the sessions, started acquiring a meaning for her with the help of transference. I encouraged the perspective of "somewhere else", a place that would be built properly, that is, without her committing some irreparable disappearing act.

She also took advantage of an opportunity to talk about her journey during two interviews with a psychoanalyst. A new dimension then appeared, around a "secret" which surrounded all her projects, and which she chose to call, somewhat ironically, a "defense-secret".

By refusing to say aloud what she had drawn during these interviews, perhaps she was able to make an attempt to subtract the object-voice, this object called *petit a* by Lacan. Recall that this object-voice had emerged during hallucinatory episodes when she was younger. The fact that she had secrets was certainly beneficial for this young girl, who complained bitterly that her mother told everyone everything. Perhaps what arose here also evoked a kind of mission, linked to the "secrecy" that the mother said she had experienced for 11 years. Perhaps this was a way of escaping the strange episode experienced by her mother when she had been a young woman. Anastasia made use of the signifiers that she was able to glean from her mother to construct a story that she tried to write in her own way, and which she was able to talk about through her personal trajectory.

At the time this article was being written, Anastasia told me that she had been admitted to board at a middle school named after a famous French psychoanalyst. She had written a fine letter of motivation, which I had strongly encouraged and supported with a letter of my own. One can only hope that this place will welcome this fragile young girl, that she finds there the means to contain the impulses that still risk overwhelming her; that this boarding school will allow her to continue to manage the right distance from her family: neither too close – at the risk of being stifled – nor too far, thus disappearing completely.

In a recent interview, Mrs. B. expressed her gratitude to those who, in the course of Anastasia's treatment, "never let them down".

Indeed, the function of the analyst is to support subjects as they build walls in order to hold on to their position in the world, to validate their discoveries and to give them the status of inventions.

References

Alberti, C. (2021). Le principe de la loi primordiale; Ce qu'il s'agit de tenir fermement à propos de l'inceste. *Lacan Quotidien*, (931). https://lacanquotidien.fr/blog/wp-content/uploads/2021/06/LQ-931.pdf

Ansermet, F. (2021, February 18). Du désir d'enfant au malentendu de l'origine. Blog du congrès PIPOL 10. https://www.pipol10.eu/2021/02/18/du-desir-denfant-aux-malentendus-de-lorigine-francois-ansermet/

Chiriaco, S. (2008). Le phénomène de la voix bienveillante. *La Cause Freudienne*, (68), 25–28.

Cottet, S. (2012). Ils ne parlent pas, ni ne voient, ni n'entendent; ils bougent. In *L'inconscient de papa et le nôtre. Contribution à la clinique lacanienne* (pp. 75–87). Paris: Éd. Michèle.

Dhéret, J. (2007). Y-a-t-il une clinique de l'abandon? *Quarto*, (90), 75–81.

Lacan, J. (1966). *Écrits*. Paris: Éd. du Seuil.

Lacan, J. (2005). *Le Séminaire*, vol. XXIII, *Le Sinthome*. Paris: Éd. du Seuil.

Laurent, D. (2021). Techno-maternités. Blog du congrès PIPOL 10. https://www.pipol10.eu/2021/04/01/techno-maternites-dominique-laurent/

Miller, J.-A. (2001, March 28). *Le lieu et le lien*. L'orientation lacanienne. Unpublished lecture given at Université de Paris 8, Department of Psychoanalysis.

Miller, J.-A. (2009). Effet retour sur la psychose ordinaire: intervention au Séminaire anglophone à Paris, juillet 2008. *Quarto*, (94–95), 40–51.

Roy, M. (2001). Enfant fétiche et phallus hyperactif. *La Petite Girafe*, (13), 62–70.

Roy, M. (2021, April 4). L'enfant, ses parents. *Hebdo-blog*. https://www.hebdo-blog.fr/lenfant-ses-parents/

Chapter 7

Franck: a case of ADHD

Sébastien Ponnou

***

The impasses of biomedical approaches to hyperactivity reveal the need for the clinic and for psychoanalysis in the care of children diagnosed as hyperactive and of their families. I will now propose to show the interest of the clinic and of psychoanalysis through a clinical presentation within an institution. The case sheds light on the theoretical benefits which underlie a Lacanian approach to hyperactivity.[1]

1. From intolerance to the intolerable

Franck was nine years old when he arrived at a therapeutic institute to which he had been sent upon notification from a French departmental center for disabled persons (MDPH) and at his mother's request following a deterioration of relationships within the family: she found herself at her wits' end. A diagnosis of hyperactivity had been made by a specialized unit the year before he was admitted to the institution, and he was being treated with a psychostimulant, which had no visible effect on his agitation. Franck had the classic symptoms of hyperactivity (lack of attention, physical agitation and hyperactivity), but with no signs of comorbidity or associated disorder. He was a happy child, at ease with respect to the faculty of speech, to knowledge and to the relationships he had with adults and peers. His academic performance was reasonable despite his agitation. He liked going to school and was involved in various projects and activities. Admission to the institute was granted on the condition that the question of medicalized treatment remain the responsibility of the prescribing hospital service. Ordinary schooling was maintained. Franck became a boarder during the week and returned to his mother's home for weekends and school holidays.

Franck's story was marked by the sudden separation of his parents three months before he was born. His father had left home without any apparent reason after several years with Franck's mother and despite having acknowledged paternity at the beginning of the pregnancy. He literally disappeared without any explanation. Franck's mother then embarked on a desperate quest to find this man, who would

DOI: 10.4324/9781003584469-8

vanish every time she located him and tried to reestablish contact with him. Franck did not know his father, nor had he ever met him.

Beyond the typical manifestations of ADHD – major at that time – an initial point of reference in working with the child was a particular symptom the mother herself had diagnosed: Franck was said to be lactose intolerant. However, she refused any medical investigation. In parallel with the standard procedures and accommodations rendered necessary by this supposed symptom, I decided to work on intolerance, with both Franck and his mother. Indeed, the difficulties at play in the mother–child relationship – which the symptom sums up perfectly – played an important role in the reasons for Franck's placement in the institution. This clinical intervention at first consisted in working with Franck on small everyday details over five years, coupled with occasional interviews with his mother. Intolerance quickly gave way to a pluralized "intolerable", which then became dialecticized and could thus be the subject of work concerning symbolization. For Franck, this meant an intolerable form of maternal omnipotence embodied in the punishments inflicted on him by his mother (isolation, toys taken away from him) – practices that the institution identified and named: "inter-diction". For the mother, the difficulties caused by her son's behavior opened the door to the intolerable abandonment that was wreaking havoc on her – that of her ex-partner, Franck's father – which served as a condensation point for a kind of untreatable *jouissance* to which she was constantly connected and of which she was the object. Franck embodied this overwhelming abandonment, of which he had become the basis, the trace and the unbearable remnant. Hyperactivity could then be interpreted as a replay of the father's flight forward as well as a means of defense that the subject used against a foreign *jouissance*, inherited, intimated by the Other and returning to the body.

The use of each one's narrative as well as open spaces through group practice had rapid effects: de-condensation of the unbearable aspects of the mother–child partnership, dissipation of the symptoms of agitation and hyperactivity associated with the extraction and displacement of *jouissance* of the Other of which Franck had taken bodily charge. Consequently, drug treatment was ceased, third-party references for both mother and child were built and the possibility of forging new forms of social relations and relationship to knowledge emerged.

2. Hyperactivity/ADHD: Lacanian signposts

Franck's situation seems revealing to us insofar as it specifies the Lacanian approach to hyperactivity (Roy, 2001) and highlights the interest of psychoanalysis and its ethics in the support and guidance of children diagnosed with ADHD and their families. In the initial situation, Franck was in the position of object of *jouissance* of his mother's fantasy. His agitation echoed "the impossible separation of a fundamentally present Other" (Cottet, 2012, p. 80). Hyperactivity evokes "a clinical movement that opposes the static nature of the maternal fantasy" (Cottet, 2012, p. 82). This relatively common position[2] – which perhaps specifies the position of the hyperactive subject – finds here its point of attachment inasmuch as Franck condenses the intolerable *jouissance* of the father's abandonment of the mother. The emphasis on the transition from intolerance to the intolerable involves the construction and sharing of a meaningful framework that allows the child to move from this point of identification to the object of maternal fantasy. Diametrically opposed to the reductionism and pure speculation of biological psychiatry (Gonon, 2011), speech-oriented treatment leads to lasting effects that enable the subject to seize upon his opportunity to create with respect to his relationship with the Other and with society.

Notes

1 This clinical presentation was first published in *Letterina*, a publication of the Association de la Cause Freudienne en Normandie with the following reference: Ponnou, S. (2020). Franck: trouble TDAH. *Letterina, bulletin de l'Association de la Cause Freudienne en Normandie*, 75.
2 "The child fulfills the presence of what Jacques Lacan refers to as object *a* in the fantasy. By replacing this object, he saturates the mode of lack in which the mother's desire is specified" (Lacan, 2001, pp. 373–374).

References

Cottet, S. (2012). *L'inconscient de papa et le nôtre: contribution à la clinique lacanienne*. Paris: Éditions Michèle.

Gonon, F. (2011). La psychiatrie biologique: une bulle spéculative? *Esprit*, (11), 54–73.

Lacan, J. (2001). *Autres écrits*. Paris: Éditions du Seuil.

Roy, M. (2001). Enfant fétiche et phallus hyperactif. *La petite girafe*, (13), 62–70.

Conclusion

Sébastien Ponnou

More than 50 years of intensive biomedical research have revealed the problems inherent in biological and statistical psychiatry applied to the child clinic. The discovery of a biological etiology of ADHD is a mere illusion riddled with unfulfilled promises. This results in the following logical consequences:

1) The diagnostic and statistical categories inherited from DSM-type nosographies are based exclusively on the coding of the child's behavior. They have no scientific reliability. Their clinical scope is limited, and their heuristic value remains highly questionable.
2) There is no causal link between diagnosis and drug treatment: the treatments currently available are nothing more than molecules or derivatives of molecules discovered between the 1940s and the 1970s during randomized trials.

Even if a biological etiology were discovered, it is not certain that it would lead to any improvement in the care, education and support of children.

Of course, the pursuit of scientific research remains indispensable: it has at least the advantage of teaching us about "what ADHD is not", and what childhood cannot be reduced to. However, research efforts can no longer be limited to biomedical research and must now include a strong human and social science component, particularly in the field of psychotherapeutic, educational and preventive practices which are recommended as the first line of treatment for children and support for families.

These limitations of Evidence-Based Medicine/Practice remind us that no human being – and certainly no child – can be summed up by statistics or the discourse of science. The essential part of therapeutic work is played out in the encounter and in the interweaving of words and the body. The child is first and foremost a subject of speech, a subject of law and a subject of desire in turn caught up in a desire that is not anonymous (Lacan, 2001a, p. 373).

DOI: 10.4324/9781003584469-9

The analyst's desire

In contrast to the distortions and conflicts of interest at work in scientific research on ADHD in France and internationally, the clinical testimonies presented in this volume highlight the commitment of the analyst to care practices as well as the strength and constancy of a desire to work that supports the inventions and discoveries that punctuate the child's journey.

Although it remains latent throughout the pages, most often veiled by the light shed on the child, this desire nevertheless makes an invaluable contribution to the subject matter of this volume: it is the necessary condition for full, authentic speech; it implies sensitivity and renewed attention to detail and to the slightest gesture; it also allows for a manner of listening that goes beyond pre-established knowledge and discourse and thus makes room for the child.

The analyst's desire is a landmark, a common thread, a mark which, together with the child's words, colors and brings new shades of nuance to the psychoanalytical encounter. But what can this desire consist of? Lacan provides a roadmap in his seminar "The Four Fundamental Concepts of Psychoanalysis": it is the desire to reveal absolute difference (Lacan, 1973, p. 248).

It is in this respect that psychoanalysts – and with them practitioners concerned with the dimensions of words and relationships – will always be several steps ahead in terms of care and education practices: they are interested in the child before and beyond his or her disorder or disability, before and beyond any pathology or deficiency. Analysts are committed to embracing the child's difference. In this way, they reject binary categories of the type "normal" versus "pathological" and shed new light on the notions of difference, individuality and subjectivity.

Individualized care for each child

This desire to recognize absolute difference is evident in the way each analyst listens to the child, his or her words, experiences and symptoms, to the extent that individuality and case-by-case work are other salient features of this volume. What does this mean? It means first of all engaging in a radical change of perspective, which goes so far as to consider inattention, agitation and, more broadly, the child's symptom as a mode of expression beyond pathologies to be treated. It also means considering that the essential process of care in psychiatry and child psychiatry cannot be carried out via standardized methods, protocols and ready-made solutions. It is different for each person. There is the child, their relationship to language, to the body, to themselves and to others, and the ongoing process of crafting so that each individual can successfully weave their uniqueness into the multitude of discourses that form the social bond. Jacques-Alain Miller even makes this absolute difference a complex universal: for the psychoanalyst, the rule is that there are only exceptions to the rule (Miller, 2008, p. 90).

This individuality is automatically connected to a dimension of invention defined by Lacan as a subject's *savoir-y-faire* with language and *jouissance*:

In a general way, if the term "invention" is essential for us today, it is because it is profoundly linked to the idea that the Other does not exist; it is profoundly linked to the idea that the big Other is an invention. As long as we accept the idea that the big Other of the symbolic exists, the subject is simply an effect of the signifier, and the one who invents, as it were, is the Other. It is only the Other who invents. Whereas if we maintain that the Other does not exist, the emphasis shifts from the effect to the use; it shifts to the *savoir-y-faire*.

It's not just the point of view that "the subject is determined by language, by the Other, it's in the Other that it happens", it's on the contrary the notion that the subject has to *savoir-y-faire*, that he has to *savoir-y-faire* with his trauma. "The Other does not exist" means that the subject is conditioned to become an inventor. In particular, he is pushed to instrumentalize language.

(Miller, 2004, p. 11)

Thus, banking on psychoanalysis means first and foremost banking on the child, and on the crafting process in which the child engages within the analytical space and which does not depend on any pre-established knowledge or routine, but rather rests on the knowledge that the child and his or her parents presume the analyst holds.

A link like no other

The desire of the analyst and the individuality of the child are connected to a place (the analytical session) and to a link (transference, that is, this supposition of knowledge that has become a request or complaint addressed to the analyst (Lacan, 2001b; Miller, 1984, 2001)). Sometimes this request comes from the child, from his parents or from the school or social system. It does not matter, because even if these variants color the scene of the encounter with their own hue, they do not make transference and the opening to the unconscious any less operative.

Transference thus becomes the link where the conscious and unconscious impasses of the subject are played out, structured, problematized and resolved. The fact that part of these processes escapes one or the other of the partners does not prevent transference from being effective, nor does it prevent the logic of the treatment from emerging in all its precision and rigor later on. The contributions in this volume, dedicated to the psychoanalytical clinic of the child, demonstrate this: an infinite attentiveness and precaution based on attention to detail and to the trivia of everyday life, what each child intimately experiences. There is no need here for proof, the scientific method or the power of statistics that are standard in contemporary discourse. Each individual case shows the analyst's style and know-how with regard to the mysteries of *jouissance* and the unconscious. Each text in this volume gives a clear presentation of analytical work, with all its meanderings and stumbling blocks, mechanisms and resolutions that punctuate these children's psychoanalytical path.

Transference cannot be demonstrated or measured: it is experienced and expressed; it unfolds and takes on various forms in the space of the session. It allows one to deal with a reality that is impossible to bear (Lacan, 1977), to cope with the unspeakable, to accept repetition (for example, that of the symptom) in order to observe the buds of a new solution. The time it takes and the way it happens are specific to each person. In some cases, the element of chance inherent in the encounter with the analyst is enough to produce lasting therapeutic effects. This was probably the case for André and Jordy. In other situations, the transition from the contingency of the encounter to the necessity of the analytical discourse requires long-term follow-up and accompaniment, which become real points of support so that the child can find his or her place in the world.

The ethics of psychoanalysis

The analyst's desire, and the notions of individuality, invention and transference converge and structure the ethics of psychoanalysis (Lacan, 1986, 2001b, p. 526). To speak of or refer to the ethics of psychoanalysis and to discuss the practices of care provided to the child start from a very simple observation: the analyst is fundamentally guided by the principle "for each individual". It is different "for each individual". Each person has his or her own unconscious, psychological life, interiority, dreams, thoughts and symptoms.

While ontologies and the great *dhommesticateurs* with universal claims privilege the doctrine "for all", morals, values, principles, norms or gold-standard protocols, psychoanalysis remains firmly on the side of the "absolutely specific", "for each individual".

Where the sirens of scientism try to impose the diagnostic criteria of ADHD to the point of being absurd, analysts devote their art and attention to the child: André, Jordy, Pierre, Sébastien, Baptiste, Léo and Franck. What matters to them is the attention devoted to the child. What happens touches on the intimacy of a subjective position, on the unfathomable decision of the being that tirelessly escapes the particularities of diagnostic categories as well as universal principles. This point needs to be clarified:

*   The category of the universal is about the whole – the notion of "for all" which is manifest in the discourse of science and most ontologies.
*   The particular refers both to that which is different from the whole and to that which remains common to the "few". In the case of this volume, ADHD is about the particular.
*   Finally, individuality is defined as that which inexorably escapes the universal and the particular: it is "for each individual".

Now, if the ethics of psychoanalysis focuses on individuality, it neither ignores nor underestimates the particular and the universal which play an important role in the social structure. However, psychoanalysts approach these particularities and universals from a perspective of individuality that guides their practice. Thus, the ethics of psychoanalysis is not antagonistic to the discourse of science, morality or ontologies with universal claims; it is additional and complementary to them, and makes a contribution to the social link based on the individuality and the responsibility of each person.

Psychoanalysis in people's lives

The texts presented in this volume demonstrate the analyst's constant concern to help not only the child, but also his or her parents, and more broadly, the troubles and pains that run through the social sphere.

Far from stereotypes and prejudices, each clinical presentation outlines the range of nuances used when helping parents in the psychoanalytical practice when they request treatment, during preliminary meetings, when listening to the child's words, during interviews, during the sessions themselves or even at the end of the treatment.

Experience in psychoanalysis shows to what extent parents, family history and the cultural and social environment constitute a symbolic and imaginary treasure from which the child will be able to find or invent his or her own solutions to thrive in the world. The children are not the problem, but the solution.

The absence of the clinic in an academic context is regrettable: this is undoubtedly because the psychoanalytical discourse has been reduced to next to nothing to the benefit of standardized tests which ignore the very existence of the subject. It should be noted, however, that for André, Jordy, Franck, and so many others, the psychoanalytical encounter was the necessary condition for them to continue their ordinary school life, whereas for Pierre, Sébastien, Baptiste, Léo and Anastasia, it enabled them to develop new ways to relate to knowledge and culture.

The fundamental conclusion to bear in mind is the following: psychoanalysis was an opportunity for each individual child to harness his or her own inventiveness, to relate more peacefully to him- or herself and to others, to master knowledge and to mature as they become – in their own way – part of society.

References

Lacan, J. (1973). *Les quatre concepts fondamentaux de la psychanalyse, séminaire XI*. Paris: Éd. du Seuil.

Lacan, J. (1977). Ouverture de la section clinique. *Ornicar?*, (9), 7–14.

Lacan J. (1986). *L'éthique de la psychanalyse, séminaire VII*. Paris: Éd. du Seuil.

Lacan, J. (2001a). *Autres écrits*. Paris: Éd. du Seuil.

Lacan, J. (2001b). *Le transfert, séminaire VIII*. Paris: Éd. du Seuil.

Miller, J.-A. (1984). CST – Clinique Sous Transfert. *Ornicar?*, (29), 142–146.

Miller J.-A. (2001, March 28). *Le lieu et le lien*. L'orientation lacanienne. Unpublished lecture given at Université of Paris 8, Department of Psychoanalysis.

Miller, J.-A. (2004). L'invention psychotique. *Quarto*, (80), 6–13.

Miller, J.-A. (2008). Le rossignol de Lacan. *La Cause freudienne*, (69), 80–95.

Index

Note: bold page numbers indicate tables; italic page numbers indicate figures.